Currents of Protection

Brian Pollo

Published by Sandiwà Press, 2025.

CURRENTS OF PROTECTION

First edition. September 17, 2025.

ISBN: 979-8232619251

Written by Brian Pollo.

Also by Brian Pollo

Hiyang: Pilipinong Pananaw ng Parmakohenetika
Hiyang: Pilipinong Pananaw ng Parmakohenetika
Salinlunas: Natural Products & Pharmacognosy
Salinlunas: Natural Products & Pharmacognosy
Currents of Protection
Currents of Protection
Resistance Rising: Genetics, Evolution, and the Future of Infectious Diseases
Resistance Rising: Genetics, Evolution, and the Future of Infectious Diseases
Phonies: Authenticity Performance Fakery
Phonies: Authenticity Performance Fakery
Biographies in Blood: The Making of Medical Modernity and Asian Medical Innovations

Watch for more at https://sites.google.com/view/brian-pollo/home.

Table of Contents

For the Biomedical Innovations Research for Translational Health Science (BIRTHS) Laboratory and for Professor Salvador Caoili

There is only one constant element in immunity, whether innate or acquired, and that is phagocytosis. The extension and importance of this factor can no longer be denied.

Élie Metchnikoff, *Immunity in Infective Diseases* (1907)

Preface

The study of blood is the study of life itself. Within its crimson currents flow more than oxygen and nutrients; they carry the histories of species, the echoes of evolutionary selection, and the chronicles of human endeavor. Coagulation, complement, and neutrophils have been sculpted across eons, yet they persist in every heartbeat, every microvascular filament, and every inflammatory cascade. To observe these systems is to peer into the palimpsest of biology, where molecules function both as instruments of survival and as vectors of narrative, where proteases, convertases, and chemotactic gradients encode not only cellular action but metaphor, ritual, and meaning.

This book is an attempt to traverse that vast terrain. It seeks to map the arc from primordial hemocytes in Cambrian seas to the programmable neutrophils of speculative futures, from yolk sac blood islands to age-related inflammaging, from complement's guidance of embryonic tissue sculpting to its destructive role in autoimmunity. It does so with attention to molecular nuance, developmental choreography, clinical reality, cultural semiotics, and biotechnological aspiration. The text is dense, intentional, and unrelenting in its pursuit of specificity, yet it aspires to reveal connections that are often overlooked: the intertwining of evolution with ontogeny, of pathology with narrative, of biochemical architecture with cultural imagination.

The triangle of blood and defense is at once humble and majestic. It is humble because its components are microscopic, often invisible, yet they orchestrate phenomena that define survival. It is majestic because they operate with precision and redundancy, a testament to nature's iterative refinement. Each chapter in this book is designed to illuminate these systems from multiple perspectives, to reveal their ancient origins, their developmental trajectory, their susceptibility to misfiring, and their potential for redesign. Readers are invited to navigate this landscape with curiosity, to observe the subtle oscillations between protection and pathology, to consider the semiotics of immune response, and to contemplate the future where human ingenuity intersects with biological legacy.

In presenting this work, the hope is that it does not merely inform but also evokes. That it compels the reader to appreciate the simultaneity of molecule and metaphor, of defense and design, of continuity and adaptation. That it illuminates the arc of life as reflected in the currents of blood and the choreography of cells, and that it provokes reflection on what it means to live within, and to intervene upon, systems so ancient, so intricate, and so indispensable.

May this foreword serve as an invitation, a prelude, and a lens. The pages that follow are a guided exploration of coagulation, complement, and neutrophils (*i.e.,* the triangle of defense) and their enduring significance across biology, medicine, culture, and imagination. Here begins a journey into the currents that sustain life and the architectures that define it.

Chapter 1: The Triangle of Blood and Defense

A single cut on the finger awakens three ancient guardians. First, the blood thickens into a fragile dam of platelets bound together and stabilized by strands of fibrin woven like a biological net. Second, a storm of invisible proteins surges through the wound, proteins that mark microbes with molecular flags, punch holes in bacterial membranes, and summon reinforcements. Finally the cells themselves arrive, neutrophils rushing to the scene, squeezing between vessel walls, releasing toxic granules, and casting webs of DNA to trap invaders.

Clotting, complement, and neutrophils are three forces that remain distinct yet inseparable. Bound by hundreds of millions of years of evolution, each arose with its own mandate: to halt bleeding, to tag enemies, to devour. Together they form what may be called the triangle of blood and defense, a network that preserves life with ruthless efficiency yet threatens it with equal vigor. Doctors see this paradox every day. The clot that seals a wound may grow into a fatal stroke. The neutrophil that swallows bacteria may also suffocate lung tissue. The complement cascade that clears infection may instead destroy kidney glomeruli in lupus.

The complement system was first recognized in the late nineteenth century, when Jules Bordet discovered that antibodies alone could not kill bacteria[1]. They needed another mysterious substance in serum. He named it complement, because it complemented the action of antibodies. Today we know that complement is made up of more than thirty proteins, mostly produced by the liver and circulating silently in the blood until triggered. Once activated, the system unfolds like a chain of falling dominoes. Three major routes exist: the classical pathway triggered by antibody binding, the lectin pathway triggered by microbial sugars, and the alternative pathway that is constantly ticking over in the background. All lead to the cleavage of a single pivotal molecule called C3. When C3 is split, one fragment coats microbes like molecular glue while another fragment summons neutrophils and increases vascular permeability. The cascade ends with the membrane attack complex, a cylindrical structure that punctures bacterial membranes. This system is as old as animal life itself. Primitive creatures such as sea urchins [2] and horseshoe crabs[3] carry complement-like proteins, showing that this was no late invention but a primordial survival tool. Yet its power can turn inward. Patients with paroxysmal nocturnal hemoglobinuria or atypical hemolytic uremic syndrome suffer relentless complement attack on their own tissues. Modern medicine has learned to blunt this with drugs such as eculizumab, but at the cost of increased susceptibility to meningococcal infections[4].

Coagulation, by contrast, is the builder rather than the assassin. It is a symphony of enzymes and cofactors that ultimately transform prothrombin into thrombin and fibrinogen into fibrin. The resulting strands form the framework of a clot that stabilizes a platelet plug. The cascade can be described as intrinsic when triggered by internal vessel injury or extrinsic when initiated by tissue factor exposed to blood, but in reality both arms converge rapidly into a single pathway. The history of coagulation research is filled with painstaking observation. Rudolf Virchow[5], the German pathologist of the nineteenth century, described the triad of thrombosis: blood stasis, vessel injury, and hypercoagulability. His insights still guide medical practice. Hemophilia, the "royal disease"[6] that haunted European monarchies, showed the fragility of this system, for the absence of a single clotting factor was enough to make minor injuries lethal. Yet coagulation is more than a mechanical plug. Thrombin also signals to immune cells, and fragments of fibrin can influence inflammation[7]. The conversation between clotting and immunity is constant and unavoidable. When balance is lost, disease follows. Deep vein thrombosis, pulmonary embolism, stroke, and myocardial infarction are all examples of coagulation's destructive potential, while conditions like liver failure or disseminated intravascular coagulation demonstrate the equally lethal danger of insufficient clotting.

The third guardian is the neutrophil, the most abundant white blood cell in human circulation. They are short-lived but numerous, the shock troops of immunity. Their armament is versatile: they engulf microbes into intracellular vacuoles, destroy them with reactive oxygen species, and release proteases that dissolve bacterial structures. They also cast neutrophil extracellular traps, webs of chromatin and protein that immobilize invaders. Neutrophils were first recognized in the nineteenth century by Elie Metchnikoff[8], who observed mobile cells engulfing foreign particles in starfish larvae. From that simple observation came the concept of phagocytosis, a discovery that earned him the Nobel Prize in 1908. But neutrophils are reckless warriors. Their weapons often injure host tissues as much as the enemy. In sepsis they pour toxins into the bloodstream that damage the very vessels they travel through. In autoimmune diseases, the nuclear debris released by neutrophil traps can provoke antibodies against the self. In cancer, neutrophils may paradoxically aid tumors by promoting angiogenesis and seeding metastasis.

These three guardians do not act in isolation. They converse constantly, forming circuits of feedback. Thrombin can activate complement. Complement fragments recruit neutrophils, which in turn release enzymes that further stimulate coagulation. The sticky traps of neutrophils become scaffolds for fibrin, anchoring thrombosis. Platelets themselves carry complement receptors, bridging hemostasis and immunity. What emerges is not three separate systems but a triangular circuit[9] that, once activated, can escalate with frightening speed (Figure 1). In sepsis, infection drives complement, neutrophils, and coagulation into overdrive until clotting factors are consumed, vessels are blocked, and bleeding and clotting coexist in chaos.

Blood has always been a subject of fascination. Ancient Egyptians linked its properties to balance and harmony, while Galen of Greece incorporated it into his four humors that determined health and temperament. The scientific understanding advanced slowly. Jan Swammerdam described leukocytes under the microscope in the seventeenth century. Virchow clarified thrombosis in the nineteenth. Metchnikoff introduced the concept of phagocytosis. Bordet proved the existence of complement. The twentieth century mapped the clotting cascade step by step and uncovered the genetic bases of hemophilia. The twenty-first century has introduced the ideas of thromboinflammation and complement therapeutics, along with the recognition of neutrophil traps as major players.

Clinical practice demonstrates the triangle's paradox daily. A patient with pneumonia may die not from the bacteria but from the storm of complement, neutrophils, and coagulation that follows. Another with atrial fibrillation may suffer a disabling stroke, a clot gone astray. A child with lupus nephritis may lose kidney function, not to infection but to her own complement system and neutrophils turning inward. During the COVID-19 pandemic the links became impossible to ignore. Patients developed microthrombosis, uncontrolled complement activation, and neutrophil infiltration in their lungs. The word thromboinflammation[10] entered the medical lexicon to describe the fusion of clotting and immunity into one destructive force.

The triangle of blood and defense is both ancient and modern, microscopic and cultural. It has preserved life for millions of years, yet it remains perilous in every emergency ward today. Blood is not only a medium of oxygen transport. It is a battlefield, a construction site, and a graveyard. Complement, coagulation, and neutrophils are its generals, its architects, and its soldiers. This is their story.

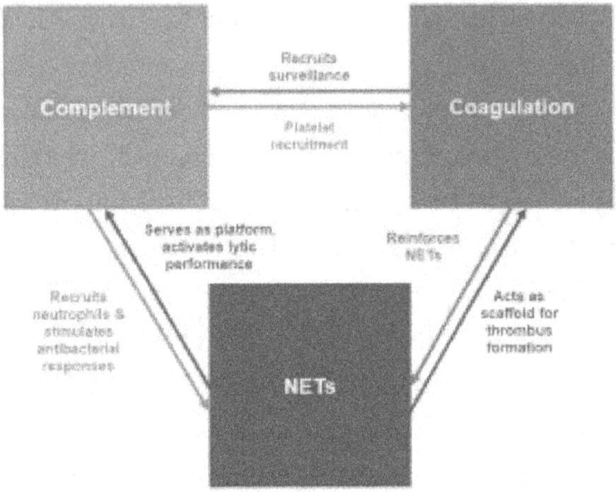

Figure 1. The dysregulated triangle of complement, coagulation, and neutrophils. Brian Andrich Pollo, 'Dysregulated Triad.Jpg' <https://osf.io/https://osf.io/axfv4> accessed 17 September 2025.

Chapter 2: Blood and Defense Across Species

Blood is one of the oldest and most conserved tissues in vertebrate biology, yet it is also a canvas upon which evolution has inscribed countless experiments in defense, repair, and survival. The complement system, coagulation cascade, and neutrophilic lineages are not modern inventions; they are cumulative products of hundreds of millions of years of selective pressure. In jawless vertebrates such as lampreys[11] and hagfish[12], one finds the most primitive manifestations of complement activity. These organisms possess C3-like molecules that are capable of opsonization, despite lacking the classical pathway or sophisticated regulatory proteins present in mammals. Lectin-like recognition molecules operate as the main surveillance system, binding carbohydrates on microbial surfaces and triggering rudimentary lytic responses. Functional assays in lampreys demonstrate that their leukocytes, while lacking granule specialization, can engulf bacteria, suggesting that the earliest immune cells were multifunctional, combining phagocytic activity with enzymatic killing in a single lineage. The juxtaposition of molecular simplicity with functional sufficiency illustrates the principle that complexity is not always necessary for survival, particularly in species with low metabolic rates and limited exposure to environmental pathogens.

Cartilaginous fishes provide the next level of elaboration in this evolutionary story[13]. Sharks and rays display multiple paralogues of C3 and factor B, evidence of gene duplication events that later formed the backbone of the vertebrate complement network. The coagulation system in elasmobranchs utilizes thrombin-like serine proteases and fibrinogen homologs that form transient clots, sufficient to prevent catastrophic hemorrhage during predatory encounters or injury. Their neutrophil-like granulocytes, often referred to as heterophils in comparative studies, demonstrate chemotaxis toward bacterial signals, though their oxidative burst is modest compared to tetrapods. Even in these species, complement proteins can mediate opsonization, enhancing phagocytosis by granulocytes and primitive macrophages. Functional integration is emerging, albeit with fewer regulatory safeguards, meaning that clotting and immune activation are prone to dysregulation under extreme stress. This illustrates a critical evolutionary principle: redundancy and regulation evolve gradually, often lagging behind the emergence of functional capability.

Amphibians such as *Xenopus laevis* provide an illustrative midpoint between primitive fish and amniotes[14]. In *Xenopus*, both classical and alternative complement pathways operate, demonstrating the co-option of ancestral proteins for specialized defense. Coagulation factors, including prothrombin and fibrinogen analogs, are present in sufficient quantities to protect against hemorrhage during metamorphosis, when dramatic tissue remodeling exposes fragile vasculature. Neutrophils in amphibians form extracellular traps under experimental stimulation, though the frequency and breadth of trap formation are limited relative to mammals. Environmental pressures exerted by aquatic pathogens and fluctuating terrestrial exposure likely drove these functional refinements. Comparative studies reveal that amphibian C3 molecules possess glycosylation patterns absent in cartilaginous fish, conferring altered binding affinity for microbial surfaces and an enhanced opsonization capacity. Such molecular modifications exemplify the stepwise accretion of function: what begins as a simple lytic protein in lampreys can evolve into a multifunctional opsonin with regulatory finesse.

Reptiles and birds continue this trajectory, presenting increasingly sophisticated immune architecture[15]. In reptiles, complement components show isoform specialization, with distinct C3 variants exhibiting differential tissue expression. Coagulation cascades approach mammalian completeness, with factors V, VII, IX, and X present in bioactive forms. Heterophils in these species are highly motile, granule-rich phagocytes capable of oxidative bursts comparable to mammalian neutrophils (Figure 2). Birds, particularly Galliformes and Passeriformes exemplify the apex of this stage, with neutrophil-like heterophils demonstrating both phagocytic efficiency and extracellular trap formation[16]. Avian complement proteins show rapid activation kinetics, and coagulation factors are optimized for high metabolic rates and rapid wound closure, reflecting ecological pressures such as predation and flight-related injury risk. Evolutionary pressures manifest not only in protein sequences but in gene regulation, with transcription factors and enhancer elements refining temporal and spatial expression patterns. These layers of molecular fine-tuning underscore the intricate interplay between environment, physiology, and defense.

Mammalian systems epitomize the culmination of this evolutionary experiment. Rodents illustrate rapid evolutionary testing, with multiple C3 isoforms, finely calibrated regulators, and a coagulation system matched to high metabolic demands. Neonates exhibit residual primitive features reminiscent of amphibians or fish, such as immature neutrophil oxidative bursts and low concentrations of regulatory complement proteins. Adults, by contrast, possess fully integrated systems: the classical, alternative, and lectin complement pathways operate synergistically, moderated by regulatory molecules including factor H, CD55, and CD59. Neutrophils contain multilayered granules, including azurophilic, specific, and tertiary granules, and can deploy extensive extracellular traps capable of immobilizing pathogens while minimizing collateral tissue injury. The coagulation cascade is finely tuned, balancing rapid clot formation with inhibitory checks to prevent thrombosis. Comparative genomics reveals that subtle amino acid substitutions, splice variants, and post-translational modifications underlie these functional refinements, highlighting the elegance of molecular evolution.

Primates, and particularly humans, showcase the apex of this system. Complement regulatory proteins are diversified and tissue-specific, coagulation pathways are precisely regulated, and neutrophils exhibit unparalleled chemotactic accuracy. Comparative studies with non-human primates reveal differences in C3 and factor B sequences that correlate with pathogen pressures and environmental exposure. The functional plasticity of human neutrophils, combined with sophisticated regulatory complement and coagulation networks, allows rapid, high-fidelity immune responses across a wide range of insults. Yet this complexity carries trade-offs: autoimmune diseases, thrombotic disorders, and hyperinflammatory syndromes reflect the fragility of a system optimized for evolutionary success rather than absolute stability.

Tracing these lineages highlights a persistent principle: functional sufficiency often predates regulatory sophistication. In species with limited ecological pressures, minimal complement and clotting activity suffice; as environmental challenges intensify, redundancy and regulation accrue. Neonates preserve vestiges of ancestral simplicity, gradually maturing into adult forms optimized for multifactorial defense. Aging organisms, conversely, exhibit the reverse trajectory, where cumulative molecular wear and stochastic dysregulation resemble primitive inefficiencies, leading to inflammation, thrombosis, and vulnerability to infection[17]. Evolution is neither linear nor teleological; it is a recursive laboratory in which selective pressures, genetic drift, and ecological demands sculpt molecules, cells, and systems over deep time.

This comparative perspective illuminates the interplay between structure, function, and environment. Every complement molecule, coagulation factor, and neutrophilic granule is a relic of ancestral experimentation and a tool for contemporary survival. By examining the lineage of these systems across jawless fish, amphibians, reptiles, birds, and mammals, one appreciates the deep temporal scaffolding upon which human physiology rests. Evolutionary insight transforms abstract pathways into living histories, contextualizes neonatal vulnerabilities, and provides a framework for understanding pathological dysregulation in aging. Blood is memory, experiment, and adaptation encoded in protein folds, catalytic sites, and cellular behaviors. To read its lineage is to witness nature's iterative refinement, the gradual accretion of complexity that sustains life in its myriad forms.

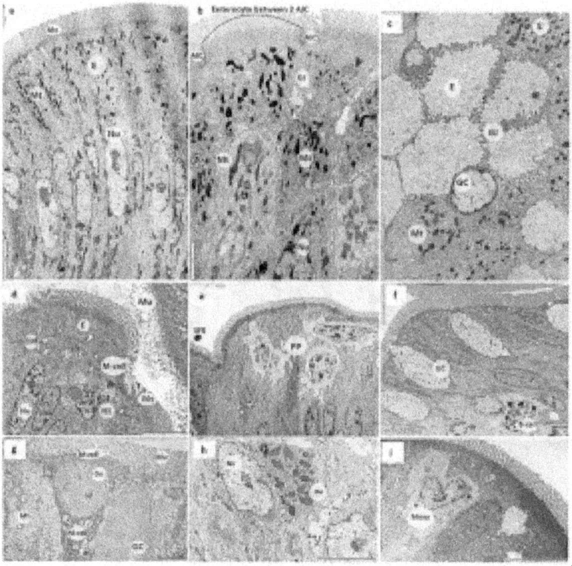

Figure 2. Transmission electron micrographs showing the architecture of intestinal epithelial cells and several types of immune cells in the ileum from 21 d old chicks. Image a is from a control chick, b and f are from a NE & H57 chick, and c, d, e, g, h and i from NE chicks. Images (a, b & c) show the ultrastructure of ileal epithelial cells, enterocytes (E), and their content: nucleus (Nu), mitochondria (Mt), microvilli (Mv) and the apical junctional complex (AJC) and gap junction (GJ). Image a show actin condensation in the AJC area (white arrows). Identified also are goblet cells (GC) that secrete mucin granules providing the mucosal surfaces with a thick mucus layer (Mu). Note a cross-sectional image of villus tip (image c) showing some light and dark enterocytes, and GC and GJ between adjacent cells. Images (d, e, f, g, h and i), show several leukocyte populations that can be found in the epithelium of the ileum, including intraepithelial lymphocytes (IEL) and microfold cells (M-cells). M-cells are located in the epithelium covering mucosa-associated lymphoid tissues, such as the Peyer's patches (PP, image e), and are specialized to sample macromolecules (antigens and pathogens) and transport them to macrophages and other immune cells to process. While the enterocytes possess a dense brush border with long, thin microvilli, M cell have apical microfolds. Image d shows the M-cell bordered by enterocytes and with an engulfed IEL;

also the presence of electron dense bodies (EDB) demonstrating ingested bacteria, while image g shows the M-cell that has engulfed an Eimeria oocyte (Oo). Other leukocytes identified are B-cells (or plasma cell) which produce secretory immunoglobulin A (sIgA) a glycoprotein transported across intestinal epithelial cells into gut secretions (image f), and heterophils (He), which are recruited to inflammatory site to clear pathogens (image h); mononuclear cells (Mono), e.g. macrophage can also migrate to intraepithelial compartment (image i). mucus (Mu). Scale bars are: a, c, d, e, f, g and i = 5 μM; b = 2 μM and h = 3 μM. Shini, S., Aland, R.C. & Bryden, W.L., CC BY 4.0 <https://creativecommons.org/licenses/by/4.0>, via Wikimedia Commons

Chapter 3: Extremophile Blood

In the remote depths of the oceans, the freezing expanses of polar regions, and the desiccated expanses of deserts, life persists against conditions that would annihilate most terrestrial organisms. Within these extremophiles, the components of blood (*e.g.*, complement proteins, coagulation factors, and neutrophilic cells) reveal extraordinary adaptations, offering insight into the plasticity and resilience of vertebrate defense systems. The study of these organisms illuminates principles of molecular evolution, protein stability, and cellular endurance that have direct bearing on human physiology, evolutionary theory, and clinical insight.

Deep-sea fishes inhabiting abyssal zones endure immense hydrostatic pressures and near-freezing temperatures, conditions that impose strong constraints on protein structure and cellular function. Teleost fishes, including shallow- and deep-living species, are known to possess multiple complement component 3 (C3) isoforms and factor B variants, reflecting gene duplications that diversify immune functions.[18] Although detailed functional analyses of abyssal C3 or factor B remain limited, isoform diversity in other teleosts suggests that sequence variation may allow complement proteins to operate under different physicochemical conditions. In parallel, biochemical surveys of deep-sea vertebrates demonstrate the progressive accumulation of trimethylamine N-oxide (TMAO) with depth, which counteracts destabilizing effects of high pressure on enzymes and may indirectly protect immune proteins.[19] Molecular studies of abyssal and hadal organisms further reveal selective pressures on heat-shock proteins and other chaperones, indicating that stress-responsive protein quality control systems are essential for life under extreme hydrostatic pressure.[20] While direct evidence for specialized granulocytes or oxidative burst modulation in abyssal fishes is lacking, the broader pattern of osmolyte accumulation and chaperone adaptation supports the view that immune effectors, like metabolic enzymes, are shaped by the unique selective pressures of the deep ocean. Together, these findings highlight that immune system evolution in fishes is intertwined with environmental challenges, though many molecular details in abyssal taxa remain to be elucidated.

Antarctic notothenioid fish (Figure 3) exemplify biochemical and physiological strategies for life in subzero seas. Their survival in waters that frequently hover around or below 0 °C is largely enabled by antifreeze glycoproteins (AFGPs), which inhibit ice growth in body fluids[21]. Genomic and comparative studies likewise show widespread molecular remodeling in cryonotothenioids consistent with cold specialization, including changes to metabolic, respiratory, and stress-response pathways. Fish coagulation systems retain the canonical components (fibrinogen, prothrombin, etc.), but while clotting clearly functions at low temperatures in Antarctic teleosts, direct experimental evidence for uniquely "cold-resistant" fibrinogen isoforms in notothenioids is limited and remains an area for further functional study. At the cellular level, Antarctic fishes characteristically maintain high membrane lipid unsaturation, a modification that preserves membrane fluidity and thus cellular processes (including those of thrombocytes) in viscous, cold plasma. Thermal modulation of immune pathways has also been documented in notothenioids. temperature influences apoptosis-related and immune gene expression, suggesting altered leukocyte behavior under chronic cold exposure, although species-specific patterns vary. Comparative genomic and proteomic work indicates that post-translational modifications and selection on protein-stability pathways contribute to the maintenance of tertiary and quaternary structure in cold conditions, implying convergent biochemical strategies to preserve hemostatic and immune competence in freezing waters.

Desert-dwelling mammals and reptiles exhibit a different spectrum of adaptation, one tuned to aridity, heat, and episodic water scarcity. Kangaroo rats, for example, maintain water balance through highly concentrated urine and tolerance of wide plasma osmolality shifts[22], while reptiles such as Gila monsters withstand prolonged dehydration by relying on water storage and behavioral strategies[23]. Although detailed studies of immune proteins in desert species remain limited, general mammalian data suggest that hyperosmotic stress alters leukocyte viability and oxidative burst responses, implying that immune cells in desert vertebrates must operate effectively under fluctuating osmotic conditions. Coagulation and innate immune function clearly remain competent during dehydration episodes, though whether these taxa possess unique structural variants of complement or clotting proteins remains to be determined.

High-altitude specialists such as Tibetan antelope, vicuñas, and Andean condors contend with chronic hypobaric hypoxia, increased ultraviolet radiation, and low temperatures[24]. Physiological studies document hemoconcentration, pulmonary and vascular remodeling, and modulation of coagulation to balance hemostasis against thrombotic risk in hypoxic conditions. At the molecular level, hypoxia-inducible factor 1α (HIF-1α) and other transcriptional regulators coordinate responses spanning angiogenesis, metabolism, and immune function[25]. Comparative transcriptomics and proteomics reveal upregulation of stress-response genes and heat-shock proteins, supporting cell survival under oxidative and thermal stress. While direct assays of complement activity and neutrophil behavior in these species are scarce, evidence from related mammals indicates that immune function is reshaped by hypoxia and oxidative stress, suggesting similar processes in high-altitude fauna.

Marine mammals, particularly cetaceans and pinnipeds, exemplify adaptations to repeated cycles of hypoxia and reperfusion during diving[26]. Their hemoglobin and myoglobin exhibit enhanced oxygen affinity and elevated myoglobin concentrations, enabling extended dives. Diving physiology also reveals mechanisms that reduce thrombotic risk during bradycardia and peripheral vasoconstriction, though coagulation protein modifications have not been directly characterized[27]. Antioxidant enzyme systems, including superoxide dismutase and catalase, are upregulated in marine mammals, mitigating oxidative stress upon reoxygenation. Proteomic studies further show elevated plasma protease inhibitors, consistent with protection of tissue and immune cell integrity under ischemia–reperfusion stress[28]. Although direct data on neutrophil apoptosis resistance in these animals are lacking, the maintenance of immune competence under hypoxic stress is suggested by their overall resilience.

Cross-environmental comparisons highlight convergent evolutionary strategies. Structural protein stability (whether achieved via amino acid sequence changes, glycosylation, or other post-translational modifications) is central to maintaining complement and coagulation function under environmental extremes. Cellular resilience, particularly in leukocytes, depends on membrane lipid composition, granule content, and stress-response pathways that allow survival during osmotic, hypoxic, or oxidative challenges. These components are integrated systemically, coordinated by endocrine, metabolic, and vascular signals, underscoring that immune and hemostatic functions cannot be understood in isolation from the organism's environmental niche.

The study of extremophile blood carries potential biomedical relevance. For example, investigations of cold-adapted proteins have informed hypotheses about strategies that might improve cryopreservation of blood products and organs. Likewise, understanding how coagulation and vascular function are maintained under osmotic stress or hypoxia in non-model species could generate ideas for managing hemorrhage and thrombosis in humans exposed to dehydration or high altitude. Observations of immune cell resilience in harsh environments may eventually guide efforts to better regulate oxidative responses or design therapies inspired by natural stress tolerance. In this sense, extremophiles can be viewed as natural experiments, offering insights into the limits of molecular and cellular performance.

Such comparative studies also shed light on the evolutionary trajectory of vertebrate blood. Across taxa (*e.g.,* lampreys, teleosts, amphibians, reptiles, and mammals) core structural motifs in complement proteins remain conserved, reflecting their ancient and essential role, whereas regulatory dynamics, granule composition, and enzyme kinetics exhibit environment-specific tuning. These contrasts provide a framework for considering how environmental pressures influence developmental processes, neonatal vulnerability, and age-related changes in immune function.

From a broader perspective, extremophiles illustrate the dialogue between molecular potential and ecological constraint. Each adaptive strategy (whether antifreeze proteins in polar fish, osmoregulatory adjustments in desert reptiles, or hypoxia tolerance in high-altitude mammals) represents a distinctive solution to survival challenges. They remind us that complement, coagulation, and neutrophils are not fixed entities but dynamic systems molded by context. Their history underscores that present-day blood function reflects both deep evolutionary ancestry and the selective pressures of diverse habitats.

In summary, research on extremophiles highlights principles of resilience, integration, and flexibility that inform our understanding of vertebrate biology. While many mechanistic details remain under investigation, these systems illustrate how immune and hemostatic pathways can function at the edges of environmental possibility. Studying them enriches evolutionary biology and suggests avenues—still largely exploratory—for future biomedical innovation.

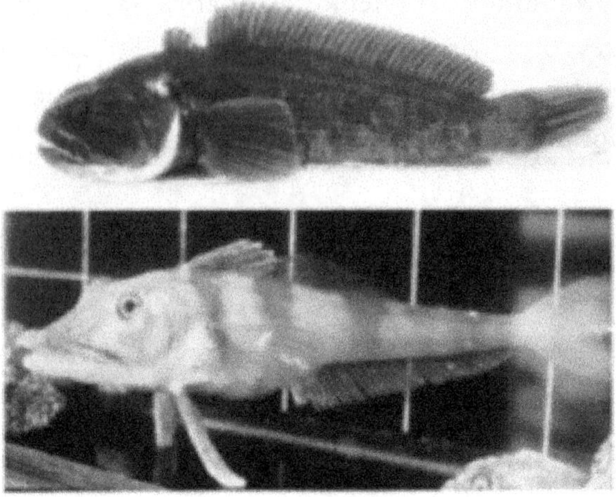

Figure 3. Representative Antarctic notothenioid fish. The Antarctic rockcod, Notothenia coriiceps *(top), is red-blooded and possesses a robustly mineralized skeleton. The white-blooded icefish,* Chaenocephalus aceratus *(Blackfin icefish; bottom), is profoundly anemic and osteopenic. Photographs provided by H. William Detrich (Northeastern University, Boston). H. William Detrich, CC BY 3.0 <https://creativecommons.org/licenses/by/3.0>, via Wikimedia Commons*

Chapter 4: The Blood Sciences Across Time

The story of blood and its defenses is as much human as it is biological, a palimpsest of curiosity, observation, and experimentation stretching from antiquity to modern molecular biology. Early physicians and natural philosophers recognized the life-giving properties of blood, though their understanding was cloaked in humoral theory, mysticism, and allegory. Hippocrates categorized blood as one of the four humors, associating it with vitality, temperament, and health. Galen expanded on these ideas, performing rudimentary dissections and observing arterial pulsations, yet still lacked recognition of the circulatory loop or the complex interplay of cellular and protein defenses. For centuries, blood was a black box, its movement and transformation understood metaphorically rather than mechanistically.

Renaissance anatomists such as Andreas Vesalius (Figure 4) began to illuminate the physical reality of vessels, heart chambers, and the movement of blood, but the notion of innate cellular defense remained obscure[29]. William Harvey's demonstration of systemic circulation in the seventeenth century shifted the paradigm, revealing a closed, dynamic system in which fluid could transport nutrients, signals, and potentially, defensive components. With circulation understood, the stage was set for inquiry into the contents of blood itself, yet the tools to observe leukocytes, platelets, or protein cascades were lacking. Microscopy remained primitive, and staining techniques had yet to differentiate cell types or reveal subcellular granules.

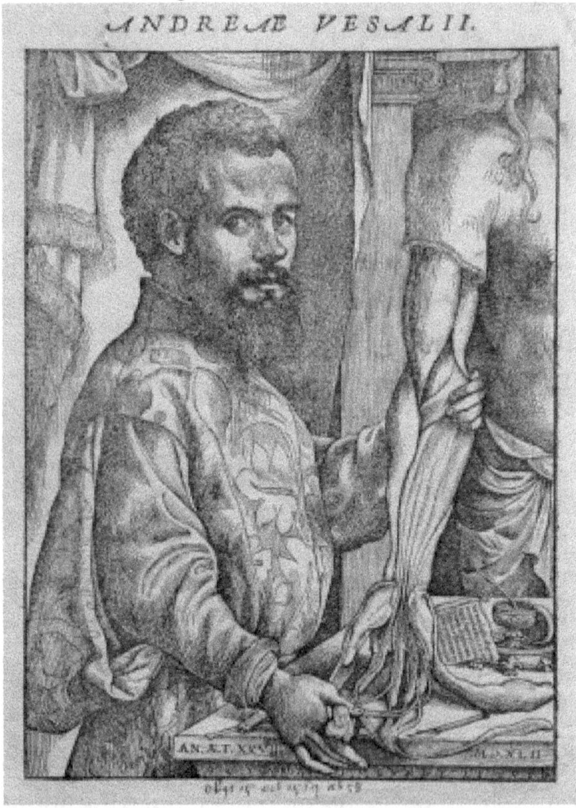

Figure 4. Portrait of Vesalius from his De humani corporis fabrica. Attributed to Jan van Calcar, Public domain, via Wikimedia Commons

The eighteenth and nineteenth centuries marked the advent of empirical hematology. Jan Swammerdam and Antonie van Leeuwenhoek observed blood cells through rudimentary microscopes, noting variability in size and form

[30]. The identification of white blood cells, later called leukocytes, suggested that blood was not merely a passive conduit but contained active participants in the maintenance of life. Early physiologists described phagocytosis as a phenomenon without understanding its molecular underpinnings. Élie Metchnikoff's (Figure 5) meticulous observations of starfish larvae in the late nineteenth century provided the first unambiguous description of phagocytic cells actively engulfing foreign particles, coining the term phagocytosis and establishing the conceptual foundation for innate immunity. Metchnikoff's work revealed that neutrophil-like cells are not static bystanders but dynamic agents, capable of recognizing, pursuing, and destroying invaders.[31]

Simultaneously, the coagulation system was gradually elucidated. Early reports of clotting focused on observable phenomena: blood that remained fluid in cold temperatures, clotted upon exposure to air, or solidified in the presence of particular plant extracts. Hemophilia, recognized clinically for centuries, prompted speculation about hereditary defects. In the mid-nineteenth century, scientists began to isolate fibrin and identify its role in clot formation. By the early twentieth century, researchers like Armand Quick and Oscar Ratnoff were dissecting the enzymatic steps of the coagulation cascade, discovering prothrombin, fibrinogen, and the sequential activation of factors[32]. These discoveries were painstaking, often confounded by experimental limitations, contamination, and variability in human plasma. Yet they laid the molecular groundwork for modern understanding, revealing that blood clotting is not a monolithic process but a cascade of highly regulated proteolytic events.

The complement system, though integral to immunity, was not recognized until immunologists investigated serum's capacity to lyse bacteria and sensitize cells in the late nineteenth century. Jules Bordet demonstrated that heat-stable and heat-labile components of serum contributed to bacteriolysis, distinguishing antibodies from complement. Subsequent work in the early twentieth century characterized hemolytic activity, leading to the identification of C1 through C9 proteins and the delineation of classical, alternative, and lectin pathways. Each advance required painstaking biochemical isolation, functional assays, and increasingly sophisticated immunological techniques. Complement was revealed as both ancient and modular, capable of opsonization, cell lysis, and recruitment of inflammatory cells. This realization bridged molecular biology with evolutionary insight.

The twentieth century also witnessed the emergence of neutrophils as a focal point of immunology. Initially described morphologically as polymorphonuclear leukocytes, their functions were gradually uncovered through in vitro assays of phagocytosis, respiratory burst, and chemotaxis. Studies using nitroblue tetrazolium and other oxidative indicators elucidated the mechanisms by which neutrophils generate reactive oxygen species. Later, the discovery of neutrophil extracellular traps in the early twenty-first century revealed a previously unrecognized modality of pathogen containment, confirming that these cells operate through multiple, overlapping mechanisms. Each insight recontextualized earlier observations, demonstrating that what had once seemed simple or enigmatic is in fact orchestrated with exquisite biochemical precision.

Experimental animals played a pivotal role in these advances. Early twentieth-century immunologists used rabbits, guinea pigs, and mice to dissect complement activity, coagulation kinetics, and phagocyte behavior. Comparative studies revealed that regulatory networks are conserved but modified across species, allowing the extrapolation of fundamental principles to humans. Xenopus, zebrafish, and lampreys later became models for ontogeny and evolution, linking historical observation with contemporary genetic and biochemical techniques. These models illuminated not only the mechanisms of defense but also the evolutionary pressures that shaped them, confirming the insights suggested by embryological studies of blood islands and yolk sac hematopoiesis.

Clinical translation emerged as knowledge deepened. The recognition that vitamin K deficiency impairs gamma-carboxylation of coagulation factors, that C3 deficiencies predispose to recurrent bacterial infections, and that neutrophil functional defects underlie congenital neutropenias, all derived from centuries of accumulation of observation, experimentation, and theoretical refinement. Physicians learned to interpret hematologic parameters contextually: neonatal thrombocytopenia, sepsis, and coagulopathy became intelligible phenomena rather than inexplicable events. The interplay of complement, coagulation, and neutrophils informed vaccination strategies, infection control, and surgical prophylaxis, translating centuries of historical insight into practical interventions.

Technological innovations accelerated discovery in the latter half of the twentieth century. Electron microscopy revealed subcellular granules in neutrophils, precise fibrin meshwork structures, and membrane attack complexes. Flow cytometry allowed quantification and functional assessment of cell populations. Molecular cloning, gene knockout studies, and CRISPR-mediated manipulations revealed causal relationships between genes, proteins, and physiological outcomes. Historical progression from observation to mechanistic elucidation exemplifies the cumulative nature of scientific knowledge, wherein each generation builds upon the labor, creativity, and curiosity of predecessors.

The history of blood sciences also reflects social and intellectual contexts. War, epidemic, and industrialization influenced research priorities, while individual curiosity and serendipity often drove breakthroughs. Pasteur's investigations into bacterial infection, Ehrlich's side-chain theory, and Metchnikoff's phagocyte studies illustrate the interplay of theory and experiment, hypothesis and observation, that characterizes scientific evolution. The development of anticoagulants such as heparin and warfarin, complement inhibitors, and neutrophil-targeted therapies reflects an ongoing translation from historical insight to modern pharmacology, highlighting the enduring relevance of foundational studies.

Historical context teaches a profound lesson: understanding blood is inseparable from understanding the people, technologies, and conceptual frameworks that uncovered its mysteries. Each discovery, from Galen's dissections to Metchnikoff's larvae, from Ratnoff's coagulation studies to the first identification of C3, contributes to an intellectual lineage that informs current and future investigation. Blood is not merely a biological tissue but a nexus of inquiry, experimentation, and conceptual refinement. Modern immunology, hematology, and hemostasis are illuminated by this lineage, providing a lens through which contemporary observations acquire meaning and trajectory.

In tracing these historical threads, one appreciates the cumulative genius, error, and serendipity that shape scientific understanding. Blood's defenses, once invisible and mystical, have been rendered visible, dissected, and contextualized across centuries. Complement, coagulation, and neutrophils emerge not only as biological phenomena but as milestones in human cognition, reflecting the iterative interplay of observation, experiment, and interpretation. The historical context is not merely a preamble to modern science; it is a continuum in which past and present converge, offering insight into the epistemic scaffolding upon which current knowledge rests. Understanding this continuum deepens our appreciation of the biochemical elegance, evolutionary sophistication, and clinical complexity of the vertebrate blood system.

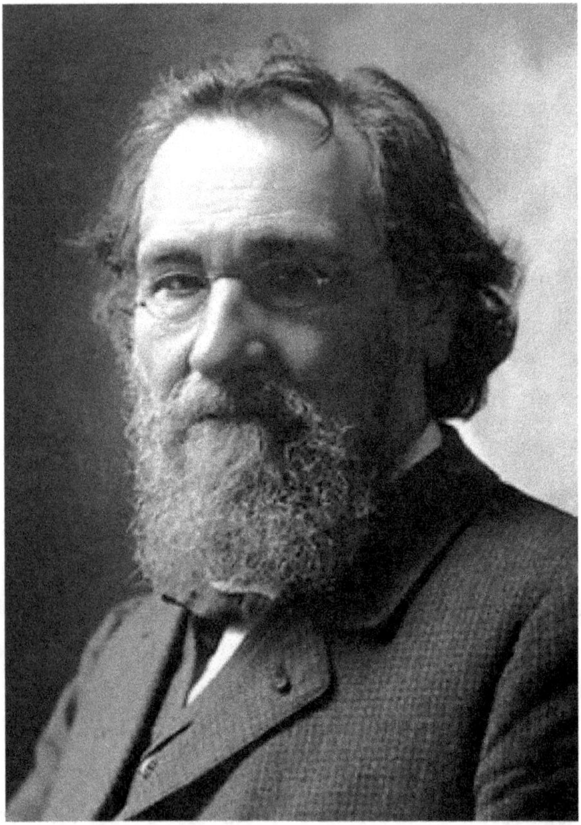

Figure 5. Ilya Ilyich Mechnikov, Nobel Prize in Physiology 1908. Nadar, Public domain, via Wikimedia Commons

Chapter 5: Folk Knowledge and Blood

Long before the molecular intricacies of complement, coagulation, or neutrophilic defense were elucidated, humans observed the living river that courses through every body, attributing to it powers both sacred and practical. Across cultures, blood has been interpreted as a conduit of vitality, a repository of temperament, and a medium through which health, disease, and destiny manifest. In Philippine ethnomedicine, the concept of *dugo* encompasses not only the fluid itself but its energetic, spiritual, and social dimensions. Healers recognized that injury, illness, or imbalance in the body could manifest through visible changes in blood, whether through color, viscosity, or the manner of its flow. These empirical observations, though lacking modern biochemical framing, often reflected subtle truths about coagulation, inflammation, and infection.

Extracts from several Philippine medicinal plants have been investigated for their traditional use in febrile and infectious conditions. Lagundi (*Vitex negundo*) is formally recognized in the Philippines as an herbal medicine for cough, asthma, and mild fever; clinical formulations have demonstrated antipyretic and anti-inflammatory activity in respiratory infections.[33] Sambong (Blumea balsamifera) is widely used as a diuretic and for kidney stones, and traditional practice also includes treatment of fever and cough. experimental studies report antibacterial effects against *Klebsiella pneumoniae*, suggesting possible indirect roles in supporting wound care.[34] Niyog-niyogan (*Quisqualis indica*) is primarily employed as an anthelmintic in Philippine traditional medicine, though pharmacological studies indicate additional antioxidant, anti-inflammatory, and mast cell–stabilizing activities.[35] While folkloric accounts attribute hemostatic and wound-healing properties to these species, current peer-reviewed evidence supports their roles mainly in fever reduction, infection control, and inflammation, with further research needed to clarify their potential in bleeding and wound repair.

The symbolism of blood also intertwined with ritual and societal function. Ceremonial offerings, often involving animals, were predicated on the belief that blood mediates vitality and protection. In many indigenous societies, bloodletting was practiced to restore equilibrium, reduce internal heat, or prevent accumulation of 'bad humors.' While such practices sometimes carried risk, they inadvertently mirrored controlled modulation of hemostatic and immune systems: minor injury could stimulate repair mechanisms, provoke local inflammatory responses, and enhance vascular resilience. Observers today may recognize parallels with the hormetic principle, in which mild stressors elicit protective adaptive responses at the cellular level.[36]

Folk narratives reveal remarkable attentiveness to infection and innate defense. Stories from Malay, Visayan, and Tagalog oral traditions describe feverish illnesses, pustular eruptions, and sudden bleeding, often attributing causation to spirits, imbalance, or environmental forces. Treatments involved topical applications of plant poultices, fumigation, or immersion in medicinal baths, many of which unknowingly leveraged antimicrobial phytochemicals. Practitioners observed that children, neonates, or the elderly were especially susceptible, reflecting an intuitive grasp of differential vulnerability later confirmed by modern immunology. The recurring motif of the "guardian within", an invisible, active agent that defends against unseen threats, presages the modern conceptualization of innate immunity, wherein neutrophils, complement, and early coagulation form a primary defense triangle.

Cross-cultural parallels abound. In medieval European medicine, leeches, cupping, and bloodletting were employed to manage fever, inflammation, or perceived excess humors. In Chinese medicine, blood (*xue*) was understood as both nutritive and defensive, circulating alongside *qi* to maintain health. Ayurvedic texts describe the *rakta dhatu* as integral to vitality, capable of transmitting both disease and cure. Across continents, the empirical correlation of blood with life force, susceptibility, and repair demonstrates convergent reasoning: pre-modern societies, lacking microscopes or biochemical assays, nonetheless perceived the dynamic qualities of blood and its role in sustaining equilibrium.

Healing rituals frequently combined observation, tactile assessment, and material intervention. Wounds were cleaned with boiled plant infusions, coagulants applied, and infections treated with poultices containing tannins, alkaloids, or flavonoids. Some communities practiced neonatal care involving protective amulets, herbal baths, and maternal blood tonics, unknowingly modulating the infant's developing hemostatic and immune systems. The timing, composition, and procedural rigor of these interventions were empirically calibrated, reflecting a proto-experimental approach. Healers noted the consequences of excess bleeding, delayed clotting, or purulent infection, reinforcing a rudimentary understanding of vascular integrity, leukocyte function, and microbial threat.

Oral histories provide insights into the recognition of neutrophil-like phenomena. Descriptions of "pus" formation, localized swelling, and rapid resolution in minor wounds correspond to the activity of phagocytes, oxidative bursts, and extracellular traps, albeit interpreted through a spiritual lens. The language of metaphor (*e.g.*, "fire within," "spirits fighting," or "blood boiling") encoded observations of inflammation, neutrophilic chemotaxis, and complement-mediated opsonization. In essence, cultural interpretations captured the dynamics of innate immunity centuries before biochemical elucidation, demonstrating that empirical observation, even when couched in symbolic frameworks, can approach objective insight.

Ritual and folklore also mediated social learning about blood-borne hazards. Communities recognized patterns of contagious illness, often linking fever, bleeding, and morbidity to proximity or exposure. Quarantine practices, avoidance of contaminated water, and ritual cleansing reflect behavioral adaptations that mitigated the spread of infection. Though explanations invoked spirits or imbalance, the practical effects aligned with principles of pathogen containment, illustrating that folk systems integrated ecological observation, risk management, and proto-epidemiology.

The resilience of these traditions is notable. Even with the advent of modern medicine, ethnomedicinal practices inform contemporary research. Phytochemical analyses of traditional decoctions have identified compounds with anticoagulant, antimicrobial, and anti-inflammatory properties, directly intersecting with mechanisms involving complement, coagulation, and neutrophils. Studies on plant-derived lectins reveal complement-activating or inhibitory capacities, while flavonoids and polyphenols modulate platelet aggregation, reflecting convergence between ancestral practice and molecular biology. In this sense, folk knowledge functions as a living laboratory, preserving observations refined over generations and offering hypotheses for modern investigation.

Understanding blood through folk lenses provides perspective on the interplay between observation, symbolism, and functional insight. Where modern science dissects molecules, ancestral wisdom observed patterns, outcomes, and correlations. Where contemporary medicine quantifies pathways, folk systems contextualized them socially, spiritually, and ecologically. Recognizing this continuum enriches appreciation of innate defense, hemostasis, and cellular immunity, situating complement, coagulation, and neutrophils within a broader tapestry of human interaction, culture, and empirical curiosity.

Blood, in this folk narrative, is both literal and metaphorical: a medium of life, a vector of vulnerability, and a symbol of human engagement with mortality and survival. The careful calibration of interventions, the attentiveness to developmental vulnerabilities, and the emphasis on observation-based adaptation demonstrate that even before microscopes and centrifuges, humans grasped the necessity of equilibrium, protection, and repair. Folklore, ritual, and ethnomedicine thus provide an enduring context for understanding the biology of blood: one in which observation, imagination, and empirical experimentation converge to illuminate the invisible defenses that sustain life.

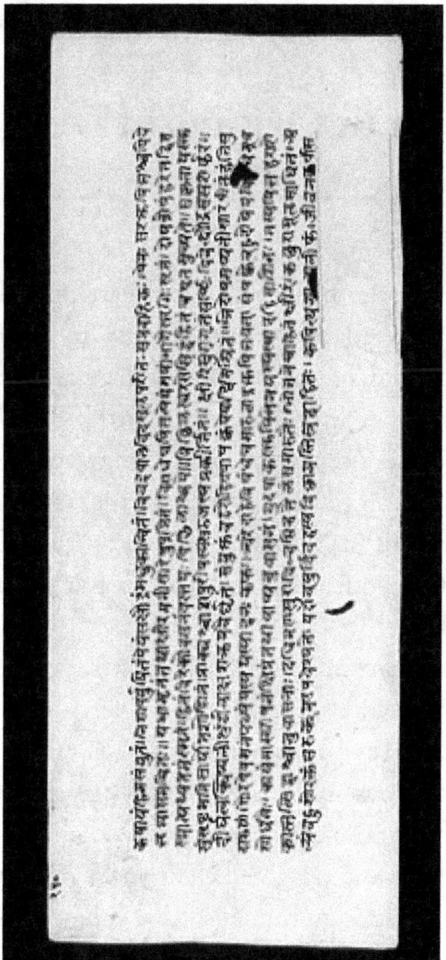

FIGURE 6. PAGE OF TEXT from the Susrutasamhita, an ayurvedic textbook, on various surgical procedures and surgical instruments. The text presents itself as the teachings of Dhanvantari, King of Kasi (Benares) to his pupil Susruta. CC BY 4.0 <https://creativecommons.org/licenses/by/4.0>, via Wikimedia Commons

Chapter 6: Origins in Deep Time

Long before the first vertebrate heart pulsed, long before bones calcified and lungs learned to breathe, life had already invented defense. The seas of the Cambrian were thick with creatures that would seem alien today, shelled trilobites crawling on the ocean floor, armored worms boring into sediments, jellyfish pulsing silently in the water. It was in this world, over half a billion years ago, that the seeds of complement, coagulation, and the first wandering immune cells emerged.

The complement system is older than vertebrates, older even than jaws and skeletons. In sea urchins and tunicates, primitive relatives of vertebrates, scientists have found molecules that resemble the central players of the human cascade. These ancient proteins recognized patterns of microbial sugars and triggered chains of proteolysis not unlike those coursing through human blood today. Horseshoe crabs, survivors from the Paleozoic, carry a clotting reaction that hardens their blue blood upon contact with bacterial endotoxin, a reflex that still saves them from infection in muddy estuaries. Pharmaceutical companies rely on this very reaction, harvesting amebocytes from their blood to test for bacterial contamination of injectable drugs. It is a strange irony that the defense of a creature older than dinosaurs remains the guardian of human hospitals.

Coagulation itself may have arisen first as a wound sealant rather than a complex cascade. Early multicellular organisms faced the same danger every animal faces: to bleed is to die. In simple chordates the coagulation machinery is rudimentary, little more than crosslinking proteins that thicken when tissue is injured. In vertebrates it became a finely tuned cascade of serine proteases, a self-amplifying sequence capable of sealing large wounds under high pressure circulation. The genetic record shows that the genes encoding clotting factors are closely related, suggesting that an ancient duplication event gave rise to the elaborate branching pathways known today. Evolution did not design the clotting system from scratch, it recycled and refined, building a network where each factor was a variant of its neighbor, like a choir of voices emerging from a single ancestral song.

Neutrophils too have ancient kin. Primitive immune cells in invertebrates, sometimes called hemocytes or coelomocytes, patrol body cavities with functions remarkably similar to modern phagocytes.[37] They engulf intruders, produce reactive chemicals, and release antimicrobial peptides. In jawed fish, the first true neutrophil-like cells appear, already equipped with granules and a short lifespan. Their role was the same then as now: immediate, non-specific destruction. It is striking that across such evolutionary distance, the strategy of using expendable, aggressive cells has persisted. The neutrophil is not an invention of humans but an ancient compromise between speed and precision.

The triangle of blood and defense was shaped by survival pressures long before humans existed. Predation drove it, because a wounded creature had to heal quickly or become another's meal. Infection drove it, because microbes have always swarmed to broken tissue. Competition drove it, because only those with reliable defenses lived long enough to reproduce. Evolution, however, is not an engineer seeking elegance. It is a tinkerer layering solutions upon older structures. This is why the complement system is not a single elegant molecule but a tangled chain of more than thirty proteins. It is why coagulation has both intrinsic and extrinsic pathways, when in truth a single efficient trigger would suffice. It is why neutrophils waste themselves after a day or two, generating collateral damage in their frenzy. These are not features designed for harmony, but compromises accumulated over millions of years.

Fossils do not preserve blood, yet they hint at these hidden battles. The armored trilobites of the Ordovician (Figure 7) bore scars of healed wounds, silent proof that clots once sealed their injuries.[38] The bones of hadrosaurs from the Cretaceous show osteomyelitis, a record of infection and inflammation.[39] Evolutionary biologists piece together this history not from fossils alone but from the genetic record. Complement proteins in humans carry domains that can be traced back to sea squirt ancestors. Coagulation factors share motifs with proteases found in jawless fish. The neutrophil's arsenal of enzymes, from myeloperoxidase to elastase, mirrors weapons seen in primitive hemocytes.

This deep history reminds us that medicine is always confronting mechanisms older than the species it treats. A doctor prescribing anticoagulants is not simply countering a disease of modern civilization but taming a cascade older than vertebrate bones. A researcher blocking complement with monoclonal antibodies is silencing a choir that first sang in Cambrian seas. An immunologist observing neutrophil traps under a microscope is watching a behavior inherited from primordial phagocytes that once crawled through the body cavities of marine invertebrates.

There is a poetic paradox in this ancestry. The very systems that threaten patients in intensive care units are not flaws of modern life but ancient victories of evolution. They succeeded in preserving life long enough for our ancestors to breed, yet in doing so they created mechanisms that now betray us in stroke, lupus, and sepsis. This tension between past utility and present danger lies at the heart of biology. Evolution is indifferent to our suffering, caring only that survival was once achieved. The triangle of blood and defense is therefore not optimized for modern human health but for ancient survival in seas filled with predators and pathogens.

The evolutionary quadrant of our story is not just about history but about continuity. Every beat of the human heart still carries complement proteins first seen in invertebrates. Every wound that closes relies on cascades that echo those of primitive chordates. Every neutrophil that dies in battle continues a tradition as old as the first phagocytes. To understand this is to see disease not as aberration but as the price of our ancestry. Blood carries with it not only oxygen and nutrients but a memory of oceans long vanished, encoded in the molecules that still patrol our veins.

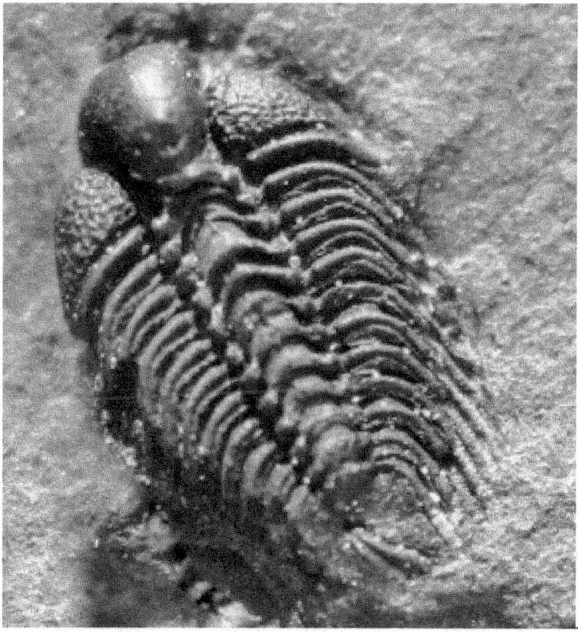

Figure 7. Trilobite: Dindymene didymograpti *(Whittard, 1960) Locality: Minsterly, Shropshire, UK Age: Ordovician , Llanvirn Didymograptus artus-Biozone. Hypostome, CC BY-SA 3.0 <https://creativecommons.org/licenses/by-sa/3.0>, via Wikimedia Commons*

Chapter 7: Arc of Development

Blood begins as islands. In the early embryo, before the heart forms, tiny clusters of cells condense in the yolk sac, forming what are called blood islands.[40] Within them, some cells flatten to become primitive vessels while others round up to become the first red and white cells. The earliest circulating leukocytes are not the specialized neutrophils of adulthood but primitive macrophage-like cells. These are the first defenders, engulfing debris as organs are sculpted, protecting against infection that may seep through fragile membranes. Complement proteins appear surprisingly early. The liver, which is the great factory of complement in the adult, does not yet exist, but embryonic tissues already produce rudimentary forms of C3 and factor B. Experiments in mice show that embryos deficient in complement struggle with normal development, suggesting that complement is not only a defense against microbes but also a tool in shaping the body, pruning synapses in the brain and guiding cell survival.

Coagulation too emerges before birth. The fetal liver begins producing clotting factors, but their levels are only a fraction of those in adults. Fibrinogen, prothrombin, and factors V, VII, IX, and X are present, yet reduced. This creates a paradox in newborn life: the clotting system is immature, yet hemorrhage is rare because counterbalancing inhibitors are also low. The neonatal clotting system is a balanced but fragile equilibrium, tuned not for adult injuries but for the vulnerabilities of birth. Obstetricians know that the transition from the womb to the outside world is a perilous crossing, and that hemorrhage or thrombosis may await if the balance is disturbed. Vitamin K deficiency in infants, for example, reveals how dependent coagulation is on subtle biochemical cofactors. Without sufficient vitamin K, certain clotting factors cannot undergo the modifications required for function, leading to dangerous bleeding. The administration of vitamin K at birth, now routine in most countries, is a simple but profound intervention that safeguards this delicate system.[41]

Neutrophils arrive on the stage with a different timing. In fetal life their numbers are limited, and their functions are restrained. Newborns produce neutrophils, but these cells show reduced capacity for generating reactive oxygen species and for casting extracellular traps. This immaturity partly explains why neonates are so vulnerable to overwhelming sepsis. Group B streptococcus, for instance, exploits these weaknesses, invading infants who cannot yet mount the explosive neutrophil responses of adults. Pediatricians know that fever is a late sign in neonates, because the immune system does not readily unleash its arsenal. The neutrophil, though present, fights with a blunted sword. Yet this immaturity also shields the newborn from self-inflicted harm. A full adult-strength neutrophil storm in a tiny newborn body would be catastrophic.

Development continues after birth, and the triangle of defense matures unevenly.[42] Complement proteins reach adult concentrations within a few months, but their regulators lag behind. Infants may therefore experience exaggerated inflammatory responses until balance is achieved. Coagulation factors climb to adult levels over the first year, reducing the risk of hemorrhage but also introducing the lifelong hazard of thrombosis. Neutrophils mature as the child grows, their oxidative burst strengthening, their granules filling with destructive enzymes, their capacity for traps increasing. By the time childhood infections become routine, the arsenal is complete.

Adolescence and adulthood bring stability, but aging reopens the cycle of imbalance. The elderly experience what has been called inflammaging, a state of chronic low-grade inflammation. Complement proteins circulate at higher baseline activity, fueling a background hum of immune signaling. Coagulation tilts toward hypercoagulability, raising the risk of deep vein thrombosis, atrial fibrillation–associated clots, and ischemic stroke. Neutrophils, though still numerous, lose precision. Their chemotaxis becomes erratic, their oxidative burst sometimes exaggerated, sometimes weak. Instead of swift elimination of pathogens, the elderly suffer prolonged infections, often complicated by collateral tissue injury. The COVID-19 pandemic revealed this with cruel clarity, as aged neutrophils and complement cascades amplified the damage in lungs more than in the young.

Across the arc of life, the triangle of blood and defense is therefore never static. It is embryonic in the womb, fragile in the newborn, balanced in youth, and dysregulated in age. Each stage carries its own vulnerabilities. The fetus must avoid bleeding before its vessels are strong. The newborn must survive infection with limited tools. The adult must guard against both external attack and internal misfire. The elder must navigate the storm of overactivity. Physicians encounter these differences daily. A pediatrician managing neonatal sepsis thinks not of the same neutrophil that a geriatrician considers in pneumonia. A surgeon operating on an elderly patient weighs the risk of thrombosis differently than on a child. A neurologist treating stroke in the aged brain understands that it is not only vessels that clot but neutrophils and complement conspiring together.

The developmental story also reminds us that biology is never frozen. The molecules that saved our ancestors in Cambrian seas are constantly being reinterpreted across the lifespan. What is useful in one stage may be dangerous in another. The neutrophil that blunts its sword in infancy sharpens it in adulthood and misfires it in senescence. The coagulation cascade that is dampened in the fetus strengthens in the child and becomes excessive in the elderly. Complement, essential in guiding embryonic tissue sculpting, later drives autoimmune disease.

To speak of complement, coagulation, and neutrophils as static systems is therefore misleading. They are dynamic arcs, molded by development, each tuned to the context of age. Blood is not only memory of the deep past but rehearsal of the life cycle, shifting its defenses according to need. The triangle of defense is not just ancient, it is developmental, alive with change, marking every stage of life with a different balance of risk and protection.

Chapter 8: The Betrayal of the Triangle

The very forces that preserve life can turn traitorous. Nowhere is this more evident than in the intensive care unit, where a patient with overwhelming infection lies connected to machines. Blood that should be a river of vitality thickens into clots that choke organs. Neutrophils, meant to be swift defenders, spill their toxins into tissue and drown the lungs in inflammation. Complement proteins, designed to mark and destroy invaders, unleash volleys against the body itself. In sepsis, the triangle of blood and defense reveals its double edge. The cascade begins with microbes entering the bloodstream, but the true destruction comes from the host. Complement fragments surge, neutrophils release traps, coagulation spreads clots through vessels both large and microscopic. Organs starve for oxygen while bleeding paradoxically coexists with thrombosis. The body is not killed by the bacteria alone but by its own frantic guardians.

Autoimmune diseases show betrayal in a slower, more insidious form. In systemic lupus erythematosus, complement plays a paradoxical role. Deficiency of early components such as C1q predisposes to lupus, because apoptotic debris is not cleared.[43] Yet once lupus is established, complement activation fuels the inflammation, depositing immune complexes in kidneys and skin. Patients develop nephritis as glomeruli become battlefields, destroyed not by infection but by immune complexes and complement-driven assault.[44] Neutrophils in lupus cast their DNA nets prematurely, feeding the cycle of autoimmunity. Their traps become sources of nuclear antigens that provoke more autoantibodies, a vicious loop where defenders provide the very targets of disease. Coagulation is not innocent here either. Antiphospholipid antibodies (Figure 8), often present in lupus, tilt the blood toward clotting, causing strokes and miscarriages.[45] Thus the triangle conspires to transform self-defense into self-destruction.

In the realm of cardiovascular disease, betrayal is subtler but no less deadly. Atherosclerotic plaques within arteries are not inert lumps of cholesterol but active sites of inflammation.[46] Neutrophils infiltrate the lesions, releasing enzymes that weaken fibrous caps. Complement proteins recognize oxidized lipids as if they were microbial surfaces, fueling chronic activation.[47] Platelets adhere to exposed endothelium, coagulation cascades are triggered, and the result is sudden occlusion of a coronary or cerebral artery. The heart attack or the stroke is the final eruption of years of betrayal, an event where the triangle acts not against infection but against the very vessels that sustain life.

Cancer adds another layer of complexity. Tumors manipulate the triangle to their advantage. Complement, instead of eliminating malignant cells, may promote tumor growth through signaling pathways that foster angiogenesis and suppress adaptive immunity.[48] Neutrophils can become tumor-associated neutrophils, paradoxically aiding metastasis by releasing enzymes that prepare distant tissues for colonization.[49] Their traps not only immobilize microbes but also ensnare circulating tumor cells, offering them a scaffold to invade new sites. Coagulation is deeply entwined with cancer biology. Malignancies induce a prothrombotic state, and clotting factors in turn feed tumor growth and spread. Trousseau's syndrome, the migration of unexplained clots in patients with occult cancer, is a classical sign of this hidden relationship. Here the triangle does not merely betray the body through overactivity but becomes an accomplice of malignancy.

The betrayal is not limited to chronic or systemic disease. Acute trauma also reveals the paradox. In severe injury, massive tissue damage releases danger signals that activate complement and neutrophils even before microbes appear. Coagulation initially saves the wounded but can then propagate uncontrolled, consuming factors and platelets until bleeding resumes, a phenomenon called coagulopathy of trauma. Surgeons know that controlling hemorrhage is not simply a mechanical task but a race against the runaway reactions of blood itself.

Even the brain, long thought to be an immune-privileged sanctuary, is not spared. In ischemic stroke, the obstruction of a cerebral artery triggers not only oxygen deprivation but also activation of complement and infiltration of neutrophils. The clot is only the beginning; the inflammatory response expands the injury, killing neurons beyond the initial core. Multiple sclerosis, another disease of the nervous system, demonstrates chronic betrayal. Complement and neutrophils participate in demyelination, turning protective systems against the insulation of nerve fibers. The mind itself is not safe from the misfires of the triangle.

COVID-19 forced the world to confront this reality in real time. Patients filled hospitals not simply because of viral replication but because of the storm unleashed in their blood. Autopsies revealed microthrombosis throughout lungs, kidneys, and hearts.[50] Neutrophil extracellular traps were woven through vessels, suffocating circulation.[51] Complement proteins were detected at high levels, their activation products embedded in tissues.[52] What was described as thromboinflammation was nothing less than the triangle collapsing upon itself, each corner amplifying the others, until vital organs could no longer function.

The betrayal of the triangle lies in its very design. A system built for rapid, overwhelming response cannot easily discriminate between enemy and host. The ancient logic of evolution required survival in moments of predation and infection, not lifelong harmony. That logic still governs the molecules and cells of our blood. The same complement fragments that signal danger cannot pause to ask whether the surface is microbial or self. The same thrombin that builds a clot cannot weigh the difference between saving a limb and choking an artery. The same neutrophil that unleashes oxidative bursts cannot measure how much tissue is sacrificed in the process. Disease arises not from malfunction but from excess, from the very power that once guaranteed survival.

To see a patient in the ward with stroke, lupus, cancer, or sepsis is therefore to see history repeating itself. It is not simply pathology but the ancient guardians turning inward, mistaking their own body for prey. The triangle of blood and defense, designed for survival, is also designed for betrayal. This is the inescapable paradox that medicine must navigate.

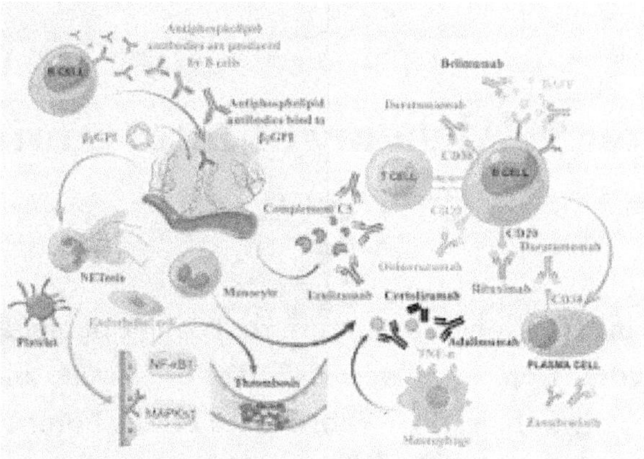

Figure 8. Summary of antiphospholipid syndrome pathogenesis and biologics treatments. Antiphospholipid antibodies, produced by B cells, bind to open and immunogenic β2-glycoprotein I (β2GPI) on the surface of endothelial cells. This leads to the activation of various target cells, such as complement cells, platelets, monocytes (including macrophages that secrete TNF-α), and neutrophils (which release neutrophil extracellular traps [NETosis]). Moreover, it upregulates the mitogen-activated protein kinase (MAPK) and nuclear factor kappa B (NF-κB) pathways, ultimately resulting in thrombosis. Several biologics have been developed to target various factors involved in this process. These include a complement 5 inhibitor (eculizumab), a type I anti-CD20 monoclonal antibody (rituximab), a type II anti-CD20 monoclonal antibody (obinutuzumab), a B cell activating factor (BAFF) inhibitor (belimumab), an anti-CD38 monoclonal antibody (daratumumab), anti-TNF-α monoclonal antibodies (adalimumab and certolizumab), and a bruton tyrosine kinase (BTK) inhibitor (zanubrutinib, which is currently being investigated in clinical trials). Zelin Yun,Lizhi Duan,Xiangjun Liu,Qingmeng Cai,Chun Li, CC BY 4.0 <https://creativecommons.org/licenses/by/4.0>, via Wikimedia Commons

Chapter 9: Alchemy of Intervention

Humanity has long tried to turn the triangle of blood and defense from a merciless force of nature into a manageable ally. The earliest efforts were crude, born not of molecular understanding but of empirical necessity. Leeching (Figure 9) and phlebotomy were once prescribed to drain "bad blood," an archaic attempt to relieve the congestion of inflammation or the stroke of apoplexy. What physicians of antiquity did not know was that the saliva of the leech contained hirudin, a direct thrombin inhibitor, a molecule of astonishing specificity. In this strange accident of pre-scientific practice lay the first hint that the coagulation cascade could be tempered. Centuries later, in the mid-twentieth century, hirudin was purified, sequenced, and harnessed, a medieval ritual transmuted into recombinant biotechnology.[53]

The story of coagulation control did not stop there. In the early twentieth century, a farmer in the American Midwest observed his cattle dying of internal hemorrhage after feeding on spoiled sweet clover. Investigators identified the culprit as dicoumarol, a natural anticoagulant formed from mold metabolism.[54] From this observation emerged warfarin, first marketed as rat poison, later transformed into one of the most widely prescribed drugs in medicine. Warfarin acts by inhibiting vitamin K epoxide reductase, preventing the γ-carboxylation of clotting factors II, VII, IX, and X. The translation of fungal chemistry into clinical pharmacology became a paradigm of how accidents in nature could be weaponized against pathological thrombosis. Yet warfarin is treacherous, its therapeutic window narrow, its interactions with diet and other drugs labyrinthine. The advent of direct oral anticoagulants such as rivaroxaban, apixaban, and dabigatran in the twenty-first century brought a more predictable modulation of factor Xa and thrombin.[55] Here at last was an intervention that combined efficacy with stability, a triumph of rational drug design.

Complement too was not immune to translation. For decades it remained a mysterious effector system, difficult to control and dismissed as too diffuse for pharmacological targeting. That skepticism crumbled with the advent of eculizumab, a monoclonal antibody against C5. Originally developed for paroxysmal nocturnal hemoglobinuria, it prevented the cleavage of C5 and the subsequent assembly of the membrane attack complex. The results were transformative. Patients who once faced relentless hemolysis and early death experienced remission. Later the drug was extended to atypical hemolytic uremic syndrome, another disease of unchecked complement activation. This was not a mere palliative but a molecular dam placed in the torrent of a primordial cascade. The cost, however, is staggering, with yearly treatments exceeding hundreds of thousands of dollars, and the vulnerability is clear: blockade of complement exposes patients to meningococcal infection, the ancient balance asserting itself again. New generations of complement therapeutics are in development, including small-molecule inhibitors of factor D, RNA interference against C3, and engineered regulators of the alternative pathway.[56] Each represents an attempt not merely to silence complement but to fine-tune its exuberance.

Neutrophils have proven more recalcitrant. Their ferocity, rapid turnover, and broad arsenal make them difficult to tame pharmacologically. Corticosteroids remain the bluntest instrument, suppressing neutrophil recruitment and activation at the cost of broad immunosuppression. More refined approaches have targeted adhesion molecules such as LFA-1 and Mac-1, blocking neutrophil migration into inflamed tissues. Inhibitors of neutrophil elastase, a protease implicated in tissue damage in emphysema and cystic fibrosis, have reached clinical trials with mixed success. Attempts to disrupt the formation of neutrophil extracellular traps by degrading extracellular DNA with DNase have shown utility in cystic fibrosis and are being explored in thromboinflammatory conditions. Yet the translation of neutrophil biology into therapy remains fragmentary, hindered by the cell's Janus-faced nature. To blunt the neutrophil is to risk uncontrolled infection; to unleash it is to invite autoimmunity and tissue injury.

Beyond pharmacology, translation has also taken the form of biotechnology. The development of extracorporeal circulation and dialysis forced physicians to confront the triangle directly, for artificial surfaces trigger complement and clotting cascades mercilessly. Biocompatible polymers, heparin coatings, and complement inhibitors embedded in membranes are the technological countermeasures. The modern heart-lung machine and renal replacement therapies are thus monuments to the taming of blood's innate hostility to foreign surfaces. Even xenotransplantation, the transplantation of organs across species, faces the wrath of complement as one of its primary obstacles. Genetic engineering of pigs to delete or modify complement-regulating proteins has become a prerequisite for making porcine organs survivable in primates. Here translation is not merely about drugs but about rewriting the interface between blood and tissue itself.

The coagulation system has also been exploited rather than suppressed. Recombinant tissue plasminogen activator, or tPA, epitomizes this inversion. Instead of preventing clotting, it is used to dissolve clots in myocardial infarction and ischemic stroke. The molecular trick is to activate plasminogen into plasmin, which chews through fibrin strands. Its use revolutionized acute cardiovascular care, though its risk of catastrophic bleeding remains. More recently, catheter-directed thrombolysis and mechanical thrombectomy have complemented or supplanted pharmacological approaches, demonstrating that translation is not only molecular but procedural.

What unites these interventions is not only the attempt to restrain the triangle but also to conscript it. Platelets are no longer only coagulators but also drug carriers, engineered to deliver therapeutics to sites of vascular injury. Complement fragments are being repurposed as adjuvants in vaccines, exploiting their capacity to amplify immune responses. Neutrophils themselves are being explored as vehicles for nanoparticle delivery, guided by their natural homing to inflamed tissues. Translation has shifted from a defensive stance to one of opportunistic harnessing, turning ancient guardians into reluctant allies of biotechnology.

The lexicon of modern medicine is full of terms that once would have sounded alchemical. Monoclonals, aptamers, small interfering RNAs, protease inhibitors, decoy receptors. Each is a talisman forged to pacify or redirect cascades that are far older than humanity. Yet the cost is visible in every ward. Patients on anticoagulants bleed uncontrollably from minor injuries. Those on complement inhibitors succumb to fulminant meningitis. Individuals receiving aggressive immunosuppression become prey to opportunistic fungi. The translation of biology into therapy is never a pure victory but a negotiation. The triangle can be tempered, nudged, or momentarily constrained, but it can never be wholly subjugated.

Perhaps the greatest achievement of translation is not in the drugs themselves but in the conceptual shift they embody. To recognize complement as targetable, coagulation as modulatable, neutrophils as manipulable, is to accept that even the most ancient systems of life are amenable to rational intervention. The journey from leech to recombinant hirudin, from spoiled clover to warfarin, from an obscure serum factor to eculizumab, from crude steroid suppression to molecular inhibitors, is a testament to the audacity of medicine. It is also a reminder that every advance is shadowed by compromise. Blood is not clay to be molded at will but a volatile element, responsive yet never compliant. The alchemy of intervention is therefore never complete. It is an ongoing dialogue with evolution, an attempt to master guardians that were never meant to be tamed.

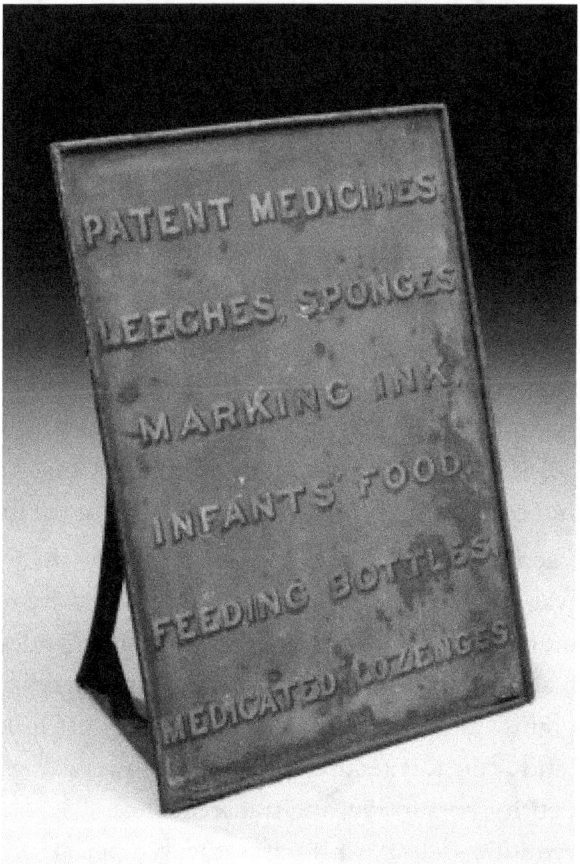

Figure 9. Shop sign advertising goods in a pharmacy, England, 1801-190. All the items advertised by the metal sign might typically be found in a pharmacy in the 1800s. These include patent medicines, some of which were likely to have limited health benefits; medicated lozenges, infant foods and feeding bottles. Like many modern chemists, the shop also stocked non-medical items; in this case ink. Leeches were also sold there. These were used for bloodletting, a centuries old practice once used to treat a wide range of medical conditions. See page for author, CC BY 4.0 <https://creativecommons.org/licenses/by/4.0>, via Wikimedia Commons

Chapter 10: Semiotics of Blood and Defense

Blood has never been merely a fluid; it has always been a cipher, a substance burdened with meanings far beyond its cellular and biochemical constituents. The ancient Greeks conceived of it as pneuma-bearing, the vital spirit that linked man to the cosmos. In Vedic ritual, the spilling of blood sanctified sacrifice, aligning the human with the divine.[57] In the medieval imagination, blood was tincture and humor, a determinant of temperament, the sanguine personality defined by warmth and vitality. The modern laboratory reduces blood to hemograms and differential counts, yet in folklore, literature, and liturgy, it retains its ineffable power as signifier of lineage, purity, corruption, and transcendence.

This semiotic density infiltrates the biological systems under discussion.[58] Clotting, in cultural idioms, becomes metaphor for stagnation, blockage, or paralysis. Political theorists speak of "clotted bureaucracies," frozen in inertia. Complement, although a technical term in immunology, resonates linguistically with its etymological kin. To complement is to complete, to finish what is partial. In ritual discourse, the notion of wholeness, of the body rendered intact against threat, parallels the immunological function of complement to consummate the act of recognition.

Neutrophils, obscure in the vernacular, acquire metaphorical extensions through their behavior: phagocytosis as devouring, extrusion of traps as ensnarement, chemotaxis as restless pursuit. Literature, when it describes swarming crowds, ravenous mobs, or invisible infiltrators, unwittingly mirrors the actions of these cells.

The anthropology of blood coagulation is equally revealing. In Mesoamerican rites (Figure 11), human sacrifice was justified by the belief that blood nourished the sun, maintaining cosmic order. The spilling of blood, therefore, was a necessary hemostasis at the level of the universe itself. Coagulation, in that cosmology, was inverted: life required not cessation of bleeding but its perpetuation. Contrast this with Christian Eucharistic theology, where blood, transubstantiated, becomes salvation, its circulation eternal rather than terminal. Here clotting is eschatological. The blood of Christ does not dry but perpetually flows, resisting the ordinary coagulative fate of corporeal blood. These cultural divergences illuminate how the same physical fluid is variously construed across civilizations.

The development of transfusion medicine in the seventeenth century brought a fresh semiotic crisis. Jean-Baptiste Denis transfused lamb's blood into a human (Figure 10), convinced that the meekness of the animal would temper the patient's madness.[59] Blood was not then seen only as a physiological medium but as a carrier of moral essences. The subsequent hemolytic reactions and fatalities did not merely mark medical misfortune; they underscored the danger of collapsing symbolic categories. The boundaries between species, sacralized by taboo, found molecular reinforcement in the immunological incompatibility of antigens and antibodies.

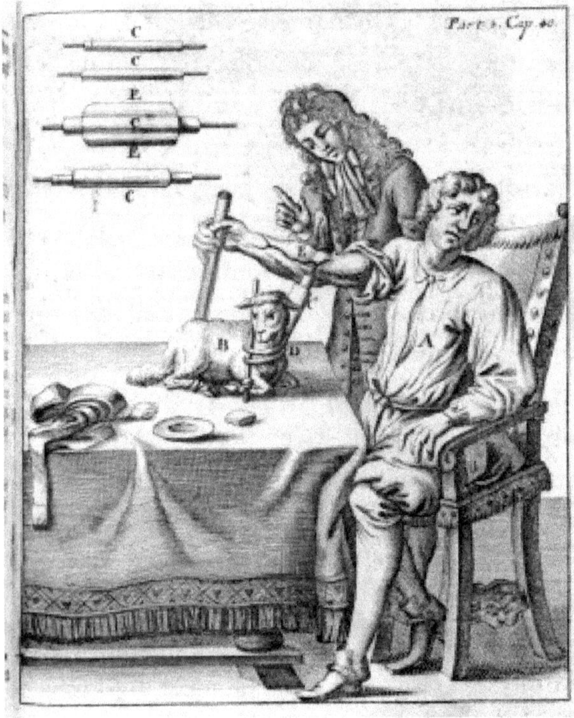

Figure 10. An early blood transfusion from lamb to man. CC BY 4.0 <https://creativecommons.org/licenses/by/4.0>, via Wikimedia Commons. An early blood transfusion from lamb to man.

The ABO system, identified by Karl Landsteiner in 1901, not only solved a clinical enigma but also revealed that symbolic boundaries were written into glycobiology itself. To transfuse across them was to risk both cultural violation and immunological catastrophe.

The lexicon of defense also overlaps with martial and juridical vocabularies. The complement system "opsonizes" invaders, from the Greek *opson*, meaning condiment, a semantic drift from cuisine to combat. Neutrophils are called "polymorphonuclear leukocytes," their segmented nuclei reminiscent of fractured shields. The coagulation cascade is replete with terms of succession: factor VII activates factor X, a genealogy of proteases reminiscent of dynastic succession. These linguistic residues suggest that even scientific nomenclature is not free from metaphor, that biology is narrated through the idioms of war, ritual, and kinship.

Evolutionary anthropology provides yet another dimension. The persistence of hemostatic and immune pathways across vertebrates has been accompanied by symbolic elaborations in human societies. In Homeric epics, wounds that gush uncontrollably signify heroic demise, while wounds that clot are signs of resilience. In Chinese medicine, stasis of blood, *xue yu*, is a pathological category associated with pain, stagnation, and melancholy.[60] The resonance between cultural taxonomies and biological realities is uncanny, as though metaphors were phylogenetic shadows of physiology.

Even modern biomedicine cannot escape cultural inscriptions. The marketing of anticoagulants is framed in metaphors of freedom (*e.g.,* to keep blood "flowing," to prevent "blockages"). Complement inhibitors are cast as guardians, preventing rogue proteins from attacking one's own tissues. Neutrophil research, though technical, borrows from imagery of "nets," "storms," and "bursts." Scientific papers, despite their rigor, employ tropes that echo myth: the neutrophil as kamikaze, the clot as scaffold, complement as sentinel. Language, far from neutral, reinscribes cultural archetypes into molecular narratives.

The semiotics of blood also extends to power and identity. [61] "Bloodlines" govern dynastic legitimacy. "Bad blood" denotes enmity or inherited corruption. "Spilled blood" legitimizes revolutions. Coagulation becomes a political metaphor for solidarity (*e.g.,* individuals coagulating into unions, movements, or masses). Complement, with its notion of completion, resonates with ideals of national integrity or communal wholeness. Neutrophils, unseen and innumerable, parallel the masses mobilized in revolts, faceless yet decisive. Thus the biological triangle is mirrored in political imaginaries.

In sum, blood is both medium and message. The clot that saves a life, the complement that tags an intruder, the neutrophil that engulfs a bacterium. These are not only physiological processes but also metaphors, symbols, and cultural motifs. Biology here is inseparable from semiotics, and the scientific is inseparable from the symbolic. To study the triangle of blood and defense without acknowledging its cultural inscriptions is to miss half its reality. For in every sacrificial altar, in every transfusion ward, in every metaphor of lineage or solidarity, the echoes of coagulation, complement, and neutrophils resound.

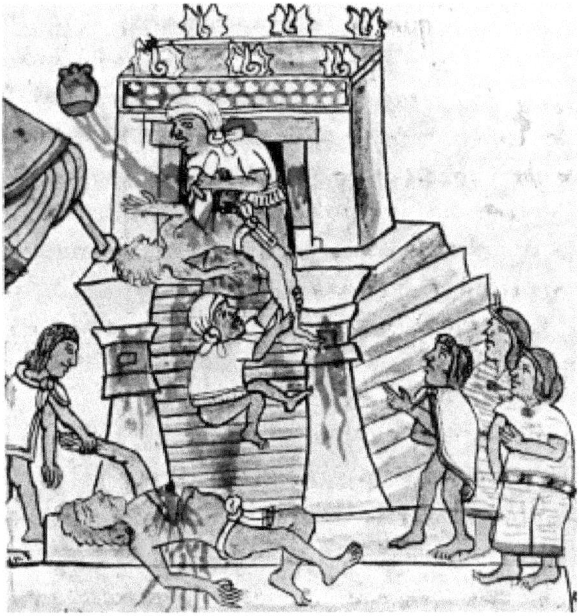

Figure 11. Aztec ritual human sacrifice portrayed in the page 141 (folio 70r) of the Codex Magliabechiano. Unknown, Public domain, via Wikimedia Commons

Chapter 11: Horizons of Reconstitution

The systems of coagulation, complement, and neutrophils are ancient architectures, sculpted by aeons of natural selection, yet the contemporary era confronts them with the possibility of radical reconstitution. The tools of molecular engineering, particularly CRISPR-Cas nucleases (Figure 12), allow not merely the suppression of individual elements but the wholesale redesign of cascades. Experimental studies using recombinant fibrinogen and naturally occurring mutations have demonstrated that alterations in the fibrinogen gene can markedly affect polymerization kinetics, clot structure, and fibrin network stability. For example, substitutions within the γ chain (*e.g.*, γ364 Asp→His) impair protofibril formation and lateral aggregation, producing clots with delayed polymerization and altered architecture.[62] Other work has explored engineering fibrin polymers through modified knob–hole interactions, creating matrices with distinct viscoelastic and mechanical properties.[63] Similarly, analyses of congenital dysfibrinogenemias reveal variants that either accelerate or slow fibrin assembly, influencing bleeding or thrombotic risk.[64] Post-translational modifications such as oxidation and nitration further modulate fibrin polymerization and clot density.[65] Collectively, these findings suggest that targeted manipulation of fibrinogen structure could in principle yield fibrin matrices with reduced susceptibility to pathological thrombosis, though this remains a future translational goal rather than a demonstrated clinical reality.

Experimental work has demonstrated that genetic modification of the complement factor H (FH) locus in mice alters regulation of the alternative pathway, underscoring the importance of FH and FH-related proteins in controlling complement activation.[66] Parallel to these in vivo approaches, recombinant FH fragments and engineered fusion proteins have been investigated as candidate therapeutics, with strategies including truncation to functional domains and chemical modification such as PEGylation to enhance stability and circulation time.[67] While rodents carrying PEGylated truncated FH variants have not yet been reported, these combined lines of research highlight both the feasibility and the potential of engineering FH-based molecules for hyper-stable regulation of the alternative pathway.

Neutrophils, once thought intractable to manipulation, are being reconsidered through the lens of cellular reprogramming. Induced pluripotent stem cells can be differentiated into granulocyte lineages, permitting the creation of bespoke neutrophil cohorts with enhanced or diminished effector functions. By inserting synthetic receptors akin to the chimeric antigen receptors of T cell therapy, it becomes theoretically possible to direct neutrophils against specific microbial epitopes or even tumor antigens. The neutrophil, traditionally a blunt implement, may be reconceived as a programmable automaton. Yet such ambitions are shadowed by the cell's brevity of life, its intrinsic autolysis, and its proclivity for collateral damage. The challenge is whether engineering can domesticate a cell evolved for immediacy and self-destruction.

Beyond genetic modification lies the field of nanotechnology, which increasingly intersects with hematology. Targeted nanocarrier systems have been developed in which fibrin-binding peptides guide thrombolytic drugs such as tissue plasminogen activator directly to clot surfaces, improving local efficacy and reducing systemic exposure in preclinical models. A persistent challenge in nanoparticle therapeutics is unintended complement activation, which can trigger infusion-related reactions and accelerate clearance.[68] To mitigate this, surface modifications including zwitterionic polymers and biomimetic coatings have been employed to limit opsonization and prolong circulation.[69] In one strategy, nanoparticles cloaked with red blood cell membranes inherit surface proteins such as CD47, CD55, and CD59, which contribute to immune evasion and enhanced pharmacokinetics.[70] Collectively, these approaches illustrate how lessons from coagulation and complement biology are informing the rational design of nanomedicines.

Artificial intelligence and systems biology also enter the scene. Mathematical models of the coagulation cascade, composed of systems of ordinary differential equations (ODEs), have been developed to simulate both intrinsic and extrinsic pathways, allowing in silico exploration of deficiencies and perturbations that would be lethal in vivo. For example, models incorporating factor XII, prekallikrein, and high-molecular-weight kininogen have been used to test how deficiencies in these contact activation components alter thrombin generation and clotting time.[71] In parallel, agent-based models of neutrophils or phagocytes have captured emergent collective behaviors under chemotactic signaling, such as neutrophil swarming or phagocyte aggregation in response to distributed pathogens.[72] Complement activation dynamics too have been formalized using network and kinetic models: for instance, large-scale ODE models of the alternative and classical pathways, with many kinetic parameters, simulate activation, regulation, and biomarker profiles.[73] Through such models, biology ceases to be merely descriptive and becomes algorithmic, its trajectories subject to predictive analytics.

The philosophical implications are profound. Michel Foucault described biopower as the governance of life processes, and in the twenty-first century this governance is molecular.[74] The clot is no longer a passive occurrence but a programmable contingency. The complement cascade can be silenced, amplified, or redirected with recombinant inhibitors. The neutrophil, once invisible in the bloodstream, can be imaged in vivo through intravital microscopy, its path traced like a cartographer's line. Control over these systems is tantamount to sovereignty over life's thresholds: bleeding, infection, inflammation. To manipulate them is to alter the conditions under which existence persists or terminates.

The future of coagulation research points toward hemocompatible materials for long-term implants and artificial organs. Polycarbonate urethanes modified with nitric oxide donors inhibit both platelet adhesion and fibrin deposition, prolonging device patency. Complement-resistant surfaces are being integrated into extracorporeal circuits, using immobilized regulators such as factor H fragments. Neutrophil interactions with prosthetic materials remain problematic, but advances in surface topography, such as nano-patterned titanium, appear to diminish neutrophil activation. In such cases, the material sciences intersect seamlessly with immunology, demonstrating that the destiny of blood systems lies not solely in pharmacology but in design at the molecular and structural level.

Speculative horizons stretch further still. Xenotransplantation, once a dream of grotesque hybridity, is now an arena where coagulation and complement dictate feasibility. Pigs engineered with human thrombomodulin, tissue factor pathway inhibitor, and complement regulators show markedly improved graft survival in primates. This suggests that interspecies barriers are not metaphysical but biochemical, solvable through rational genomic grafting. The philosophical boundary between human and non-human is being rewritten in coagulation factors and complement proteins. Neutrophils, with their aggressive recognition of non-self, remain obstacles, but strategies that induce tolerance or transient suppression may overcome their intransigence.

Even more radical is the idea of synthetic blood, an aspiration pursued for decades with perfluorocarbon emulsions and hemoglobin-based oxygen carriers. These substitutes, while focused on gas transport, inevitably confront coagulation and complement, for no fluid can circulate without awakening these systems. Recent efforts use microfluidic platforms to emulate the rheology of capillary beds, testing whether artificial suspensions can traverse without triggering clotting or immune activation. If successful, synthetic blood would not merely replace a component of physiology but rewrite the ecology of circulation itself, altering how coagulation, complement, and neutrophils recognize the very substance they patrol.

The cultural imagination has not lagged behind. In speculative fiction, post-human entities possess self-healing circulations in which coagulation occurs instantaneously without thrombosis, complement adapts dynamically to novel pathogens, and neutrophils function as semi-autonomous drones. While fantastical, these visions gesture toward trajectories already unfolding in laboratories. What is imagined in narrative form is often prototyped in molecular engineering, a feedback loop between imagination and experiment.

Ultimately the horizon of reconstitution reveals that blood's systems are not immutable legacies but mutable infrastructures. They are open to editing, augmentation, and replacement. Yet the risks are as formidable as the promises. To alter coagulation risks hemorrhage or occlusion. To silence complement risks infection or unchecked proliferation. To manipulate neutrophils risks unleashing tissue destruction. The future will therefore not abolish the triangle of blood and defense but render it plastic, negotiable, and perpetually in flux.

Blood, once sacred, once feared, once dissected, is now being rewritten. It is not only a fluid of survival but a text of possibility, each clot, each cascade, each swarm of neutrophils a syllable in an evolving grammar. The horizon does not promise transcendence but reconstitution, a future where the systems that once defined life's limits become subjects of authorship.

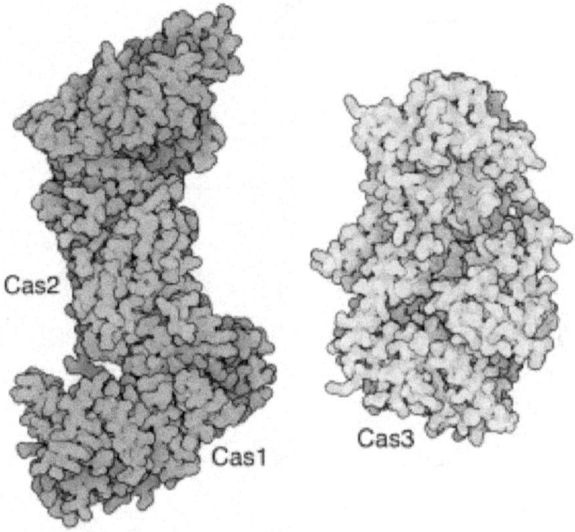

Figure 12. Space-filled drawings of Cas (CRISPR-associated) proteins of the CRISPR bacterial immune system. At left is a complex of the Cas1 and Cas2 proteins which cleave the right length guide pieces of RNA from an initial virus infection for storage in the CRISPR genomic archive. At right is Cas3, the "executioner" enzyme that chops up the invading DNA from a later invasion of the same virus, when it has been recognized by the Cascade complex. Drawn by David Goodsell from PDB entries 4p6i and 4qqw. David Goodsell, CC BY 3.0 <https://creativecommons.org/licenses/by/3.0>, via Wikimedia Commons

Chapter 12: Convergence of Epochs

The triangle of blood and defense is at once ancient and immediate, microscopic and cosmic, corporeal and semiotic. To apprehend its totality requires traversing deep time, embryonic genesis, clinical catastrophe, cultural codification, and speculative redesign. Each domain is a lens, each lens refracts the same elemental forces: fibrin polymerization, proteolytic cascades, opsonization, chemotaxis, degranulation, and the ephemeral choreography of neutrophils. Evolution left traces in the sequences of complement proteins, the duplicated serine proteases, the segmented nuclei of granulocytes, yet it also inscribed these traces into ontogeny, pathology, and the human imagination.

In evolutionary terms, the persistence of factor C3 across chordates and the conservation of neutrophil-like hemocytes in echinoderms underscores the robustness of these systems. The selective pressures of predation, microbial colonization, and hemorrhagic risk shaped them into circuits capable of immediate amplification. Yet redundancy is their hallmark. Paralogs, isoforms, and alternative pathways proliferate not as extravagance but as contingency. The alternative, classical, and lectin complement pathways form a triad of surveillance, much like the multiple coagulation pathways that permit thrombin generation even when extrinsic or intrinsic factors falter. This redundancy, while adaptive in primordial seas, manifests as fragility in modern disease, where excess and misfiring become pathology.

Developmental biology reveals the temporal choreography of these systems. Fetal expression of complement components precedes hepatic maturation, with C1q and factor B detectable in extrahepatic sites. The neonatal coagulation system balances procoagulant and anticoagulant forces in a delicate equilibrium, reliant on vitamin K–dependent gamma-carboxylation and maternal nutrient transfer. Neutrophils mature postnatally, their chemotactic responsiveness and oxidative burst capacity gradually approaching adult phenotypes. This developmental staging explains neonatal susceptibility to septicemia and intraventricular hemorrhage, while also highlighting the intricate interplay between ontogeny and evolutionary heritage.

Pathology demonstrates the peril of misregulated power. Sepsis, systemic lupus erythematosus, thromboembolic disorders, ischemic stroke, and malignancy illustrate how the triangle of blood and defense, when untempered, transforms from protector into assassin. Complement fragments deposit in glomeruli, neutrophil extracellular traps occlude microvasculature, and coagulation cascades propagate intravascular thrombi. The clinical tableaux are vivid: kidneys congested with fibrin, lungs suffused with neutrophilic debris, coronary arteries occluded by platelets enmeshed in fibrin lattices. The betrayal is not aberrant; it is an amplification of evolutionary strategies optimized for rapid response and survival rather than long-term equilibrium.

Translation, the domain of human intervention, demonstrates both ingenuity and hubris. Hirudin, warfarin, eculizumab, recombinant tissue plasminogen activator, neutrophil elastase inhibitors, and DNase therapies exemplify our capacity to manipulate these systems. Nanotechnology, intravital imaging, synthetic scaffolds, and CRISPR-mediated reprogramming extend control into previously inaccessible domains. Each manipulation is informed by computational modeling, pharmacokinetics, and bioengineering, yet every intervention invokes risk. Hemorrhage, infection, thrombosis, and immune dysregulation are constant companions. In our laboratories, the triangle is both subject and object, a material to be sculpted, a system to be negotiated.

Cultural semiotics contextualize this biology in human consciousness. Blood, in its metaphoric and ritual dimensions, encodes lineage, vitality, sanctity, and aggression. Coagulation is stasis and solidarity, complement is completion and defense, neutrophils are devouring masses or sacrificial intermediaries. The narratives humans construct around blood echo its molecular imperatives. Sacrifice, transfusion, ritual purification, and heroic wounding are not arbitrary; they are cultural reflections of processes that are themselves selective, destructive, and regenerative. The semiotic overlay illuminates the reciprocal influence of biology and meaning, showing how scientific discourse and cultural metaphor are entangled.

Speculative futures extend the convergence beyond the present. CRISPR-edited coagulation factors, neutrophils with synthetic chemotactic receptors, complement regulators fused to polymer scaffolds, hemocompatible implants, and engineered erythrocyte-mimetic nanoparticles redefine the landscape. These interventions illustrate a transhuman horizon where mortality, infection, thrombosis, and inflammation may be partially scripted, where biological contingencies can be engineered for precision. Philosophically, this invokes questions of biopower, agency, and the ethics of editing systems honed over hundreds of millions of years. Each engineered alteration is a negotiation with evolutionary logic, a conversation with history, a wager with the stochastic forces that govern life and death.

Taken together, the triangle of blood and defense is a prism through which the entirety of biology, medicine, culture, and technology can be viewed. Its evolution teaches robustness and redundancy, its development instructs timing and balance, its pathology warns of power untempered, its translation exemplifies intervention and design, its cultural resonance reveals symbolism and semiotics, and its future intimates the possibility of authorship over life's fundamental arbiters. The triangle is not merely a system; it is a narrative, a recurring motif in the chronicle of life, a cipher whose interpretation spans aeons.

As humans confront the triangle with scalpel, needle, and nucleotide, they inherit both its gifts and its curses. Blood carries oxygen, nutrients, and immunity, but also memory, risk, and semiotic weight. Clotting seals wounds yet harbors thrombotic potential. Complement protects yet destroys. Neutrophils defend yet devastate. The convergence of these forces within individuals and populations illustrates the paradox of survival: the same systems that allow life to flourish can also precipitate its collapse. Understanding the triangle in its full dimensionality (*i.e.,* temporal, molecular, clinical, cultural, and technological) is the prerequisite not for mastery but for negotiation, not for absolute control but for coexistence with the elemental architectures of life.

In the final reckoning, the triangle of blood and defense is both inheritance and responsibility, a testament to the resilience of life and a reminder of its fragility. Each pulse, each clot, each cascade is a dialogue between history and present, between molecules and meaning, between human intention and evolutionary design. It is in this dialogue that the essence of blood and immunity, coagulation and phagocytosis, complement and neutrophil, is inscribed, not only in the body but in the very consciousness that contemplates it.

Epilogue: Codex of Circulation

Blood flows not only as a medium of life but as a codex of existence, a living manuscript in which the chronicles of evolution, development, pathology, culture, and future design are inscribed. Every erythrocyte carries not merely oxygen but a palimpsest of genetic history. Every neutrophil, every fibrin strand, every complement fragment is a lexeme in a biochemical script that has endured the eons, a testament to selective pressures that shaped vertebrate immunity. Hemostasis, inflammation, and cellular recognition are not isolated phenomena but integrated epistles, their syntax governed by proteases, cofactors, chemotactic gradients, and signalosomes whose interactions have been honed for survival and reproduction.

The evolutionary substratum of this codex is palpable in the conservation of serpins, thrombospondins, and C-type lectins across taxa. Sea lampreys and hagfish, ancient agnathans, deploy coagulation-like mechanisms through primitive prothrombin analogues and clot-forming glycoproteins, demonstrating that the architecture of defense predates jaws and adaptive immunity. The emergence of polymorphonuclear granulocytes in gnathostomes marked a critical inflection point, a cellular specialization that permitted rapid microbial neutralization while maintaining vascular integrity. Complement orthologs, including C3 and factor B, are expressed in teleosts and elasmobranchs, their sequence homology revealing a molecular dialogue that spans hundreds of millions of years.

Ontogeny mirrors phylogeny in remarkable ways. Fetal hepatic stellate cells, yolk sac-derived macrophages, and embryonic neutrophil progenitors choreograph a temporal ballet in which complement and coagulation factors appear in staged sequences. The neonate exhibits a milieu of hypocoagulable factors tempered by underdeveloped inhibitors, a condition balanced by maternal-fetal transfers of immunoglobulins and vitamin K–dependent factors. Chemotactic gradients and cytokine milieu modulate neutrophil maturation, preparing the infant for the microbial challenges of ex utero existence. This developmental calibration illustrates that each stage of life is a negotiation between genetic heritage, environmental exposure, and biochemical contingency.

Pathology illustrates the cataclysmic potential of misalignment. Disseminated intravascular coagulation, catastrophic antiphospholipid syndrome, necrotizing fasciitis, and hyperinflammatory syndromes exemplify scenarios in which the triangle betrays the host. Complement deposition in glomeruli, neutrophil extracellular trap entanglement of capillaries, and fibrin occlusion of microvasculature converge to precipitate organ failure. The stochasticity inherent in these cascades means that minor perturbations (*e.g.*, an obscure polymorphism, a transient infection, a dietary deficiency) can initiate a chain reaction culminating in systemic catastrophe. Clinical management requires a balance of anticoagulation, immunomodulation, and supportive care, reflecting both the sophistication and fragility of intervention.

Translation into therapeutics is an ongoing exercise in biomolecular diplomacy. Recombinant anticoagulants, aptamer-based complement inhibitors, neutrophil chemotaxis modulators, and intravital imaging-guided interventions exemplify humanity's capacity to modulate ancient circuits. The deployment of factor XIII stabilizers, MASP inhibitors, and nanoparticle cloaks for synthetic blood illustrates the intersection of engineering and physiology. These interventions are not neutral; they rewrite the codex, selectively enhancing or suppressing specific pathways, a practice reminiscent of alchemical transmutation yet grounded in biophysical precision. The risk-benefit calculus is intricate. Hypercoagulability must be restrained without inducing hemorrhage. Complement inhibition must forestall autoimmune damage without inviting sepsis. Neutrophil modulation must reduce collateral injury without compromising microbial defense. Each therapeutic decision is a microcosm of evolutionary negotiation, a dialogue between intervention and natural design.

Cultural interpretation persists alongside molecular understanding. Blood remains an icon of vitality and lineage. Rituals of scarification, transfusion ceremonies, and sacrificial rites encode social hierarchies, cosmological beliefs, and moral imperatives. Clotting metaphors permeate discourse: bloodlines, stagnation, and fluidity inform social, political, and literary frameworks. Complement and neutrophils, while less visible, inspire allegories of guardianship, vigilance, and collective action. The interplay between biology and semiotics demonstrates that human cognition constantly interprets molecular reality through narrative and symbol, revealing that understanding of physiology is inseparable from cultural cognition.

The speculative horizon extends these narratives into a post-human paradigm. Genomic reconfiguration through CRISPR, synthetic hematology, organ-on-chip modeling, and nanostructured biomimetic surfaces render the triangle malleable. Designer neutrophils with programmable chemotaxis, complement regulators fused to recombinant scaffolds, and thrombin analogues with adjustable kinetics are conceivable interventions. In silico modeling predicts outcomes with unprecedented fidelity, yet stochasticity, epistasis, and environmental flux remain intractable variables. Philosophically, this raises questions of agency, authorship, and ethics: to what extent should humans assume dominion over systems refined across geologic epochs? The codex of circulation is no longer merely observed; it is authored, edited, and annotated, its evolutionary voice complemented by human ingenuity.

The triangle, when synthesized across epochs, emerges as a metaphor for the human condition. Survival requires rapid response, calculated modulation, cultural codification, and forward-looking innovation. Each fibrin filament, complement fragment, and neutrophil swarm is simultaneously a product of selection, a vector of disease, a target of intervention, and a symbol of meaning. Life persists because of these systems and is endangered because of them, their duality mirrored in human cognition and society. To study them is to confront the paradox of vitality: the same circuits that sustain existence can precipitate demise, the same molecules that defend can destroy, the same cells that nurture can betray.

In closing, the triangle of blood and defense is a manuscript continuously written, interpreted, and reinterpreted. It spans molecular genetics, embryology, clinical pathology, cultural semiotics, and speculative biotechnology. It embodies temporal continuity, from Cambrian hemocytes to futuristic synthetic circulations. It is both inheritance and responsibility, demanding respect, comprehension, and careful negotiation. Humanity's interaction with this triangle is a microcosm of its broader engagement with nature: an endeavor to understand, to harness, to reinterpret, and ultimately to coexist with forces far older and more intricate than consciousness alone can dictate. The codex of circulation remains open, each pulse a line of verse, each cascade a stanza, each intervention a footnote in the evolving anthology of life.

Index

Sandiwà Publishing is an independent press devoted to works that unite spirit (diwà) and intellect. Its catalogue bridges creative nonfiction, ethnomedicine, history, and the sciences, reflecting the conviction that knowledge is strongest when culture and inquiry walk together. Each publication honors heritage while engaging the challenges of the present, affirming that literature can be both an archive of memory and a spark for new ideas.

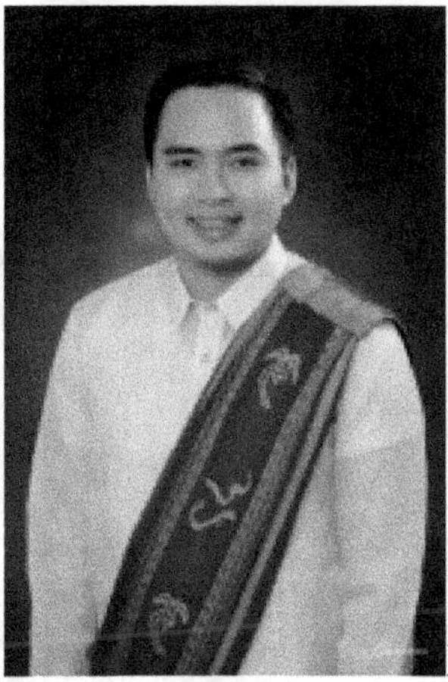

Brian Pollo is an MD-PhD candidate, educator, and writer whose work spans biochemistry, ethnomedicine, and the history of science. They study how complement, coagulation, and innate immunity adapt in extreme environments, while also tracing the cultural and symbolic roles of blood in human storytelling. Their writing blends scientific rigor with narrative inquiry, reflecting a commitment to both biomedical innovation and the preservation of ancestral knowledge.

[1] Jean Marc Cavaillon, Philippe Sansonetti and Michel Goldman, '[Jules Bordet, a Man of Conviction. Centenary of His Nobel Prize]' (2020) 36 Medecine sciences: M/S 803 <https://pubmed.ncbi.nlm.nih.gov/32821055/> accessed 17 September 2025; Jean Marc Cavaillon, Philippe Sansonetti and Michel Goldman, '100th Anniversary of Jules Bordet's Nobel Prize: Tribute to a Founding Father of Immunology' (2019) 10 Frontiers in immunology <https://pubmed.ncbi.nlm.nih.gov/31572361/> accessed 17 September 2025.

[2] L Courtney Smith, Lori A Clow and David P Terwilliger, 'The Ancestral Complement System in Sea Urchins' (2001) 180 Immunological reviews 16 <https://pubmed.ncbi.nlm.nih.gov/11414357/> accessed 17 September 2025; Julie Ghosh and others, 'Invertebrate Immune Diversity' (2011) 35 Developmental and Comparative Immunology 959 <https://pubmed.ncbi.nlm.nih.gov/21182860/> accessed 17 September 2025.

[3] Shun Ichiro Kawabata and Ryoko Tsuda, 'Molecular Basis of Non-Self Recognition by the Horseshoe Crab Tachylectins' (2002) 1572 Biochimica et Biophysica Acta - General Subjects 414 <https://pubmed.ncbi.nlm.nih.gov/12223283/> accessed 17 September 2025.

[4] Jeroen D Langereis and others, 'Eculizumab Impairs Neisseria Meningitidis Serogroup B Killing in Whole Blood despite 4CMenB Vaccination of PNH Patients' (2020) 4 Blood advances 3615 <https://pubmed.ncbi.nlm.nih.gov/32766853/> accessed 17 September 2025.

[5] Sam Safavi-Abbasi and others, 'Rudolf Ludwig Karl Virchow: Pathologist, Physician, Anthropologist, and Politician. Implications of His Work for the Understanding of Cerebrovascular Pathology and Stroke' (2006) 20 Neurosurgical focus 1 <https://pubmed.ncbi.nlm.nih.gov/16819807/> accessed 17 September 2025.

[6] P Green, 'The "Royal Disease"' (2010) 8 Journal of Thrombosis and Haemostasis 2214 <https://pubmed.ncbi.nlm.nih.gov/20670371/> accessed 17 September 2025.

[7] Sergiy Yakovlev, Dudley K Strickland and Leonid Medved, 'Current View on the Molecular Mechanisms Underlying Fibrin(Ogen)-Dependent Inflammation' (2022) 122 Thrombosis and haemostasis 1858 <https://pubmed.ncbi.nlm.nih.gov/35896433/> accessed 17 September 2025.

[8] Charlotte R Edwards and Peter E Lipsky, 'How Does Elie Metchnikoff Relate to the Investigator of Today?' [2025] Annals of the rheumatic diseases <https://pubmed.ncbi.nlm.nih.gov/40754488/> accessed 17 September 2025.

[9] Cynthia M de Bont, Wilbert C Boelens and Ger JM Pruijn, 'NETosis, Complement, and Coagulation: A Triangular Relationship' (2019) 16 Cellular & molecular immunology 19 <https://pubmed.ncbi.nlm.nih.gov/29572545/> accessed 17 September 2025.

[10] Denisa D Wagner and Lukas A Heger, 'Thromboinflammation: From Atherosclerosis to COVID-19' (2022) 42 Arteriosclerosis, thrombosis, and vascular biology 1103 <https://pubmed.ncbi.nlm.nih.gov/35861953/> accessed 17 September 2025.

[11] Misao Matsushita, 'The Complement System of Agnathans' (2018) 9 Frontiers in immunology <https://pubmed.ncbi.nlm.nih.gov/29967624/> accessed 17 September 2025.

[12] Tomokazu Yamaguchi and others, 'Hagfish C1q: Its Unique Binding Property' (2014) 43 Developmental and Comparative Immunology 47 <https://pubmed.ncbi.nlm.nih.gov/24201131/> accessed 17 September 2025.

[13] Masaru Nonaka and Sylvia L Smith, 'Complement System of Bony and Cartilaginous Fish' (2000) 10 Fish & shellfish immunology 215 <https://pubmed.ncbi.nlm.nih.gov/10938735/> accessed 17 September 2025.

[14] Fangfang Yan and others, 'Complement C1q Subunit Molecules from Xenopus Laevis Possess Conserved Function in C1q-Immunoglobulin Interaction' (2020) 103 Developmental and

comparative immunology <https://pubmed.ncbi.nlm.nih.gov/31678076/> accessed 17 September 2025.

[15] Praveen Papareddy and others, 'An Ecoimmunological Approach to Study Evolutionary and Ancient Links between Coagulation, Complement and Innate Immunity' (2018) 9 Virulence 724 <https://pubmed.ncbi.nlm.nih.gov/29473457/> accessed 17 September 2025.

[16] Kenneth J Genovese and others, 'The Avian Heterophil' (2013) 41 Developmental and Comparative Immunology 334 <https://pubmed.ncbi.nlm.nih.gov/23583524/> accessed 17 September 2025.

[17] Runzi Zheng and others, 'The Complement System, Aging, and Aging-Related Diseases' (2022) 23 International journal of molecular sciences <https://pubmed.ncbi.nlm.nih.gov/35955822/> accessed 17 September 2025.

[18] J Oriol Sunyer, Lluis Tort and John D Lambris, 'Diversity of the Third Form of Complement, C3, in Fish: Functional Characterization of Five Forms of C3 in the Diploid Fish Sparus Aurata' (1997) 326 Biochemical Journal 877; Gabriel Forn-Cuní and others, 'The Evolution and Appearance of C3 Duplications in Fish Originate an Exclusive Teleost C3 Gene Form with Anti-Inflammatory Activity' (2014) 9 PLoS ONE e99673 <https://pmc.ncbi.nlm.nih.gov/articles/PMC4057122/> accessed 17 September 2025; M Claire H Holland and John D Lambris, 'The Complement System in Teleosts' (2002) 12 Fish and Shellfish Immunology 399 <https://pubmed.ncbi.nlm.nih.gov/12194452/> accessed 17 September 2025.

[19] Paul H Yancey and others, 'Marine Fish May Be Biochemically Constrained from Inhabiting the Deepest Ocean Depths' (2014) 111 Proceedings of the National Academy of Sciences of the United States of America 4461 <https://pmc.ncbi.nlm.nih.gov/articles/PMC3970477/> accessed 17 September 2025.

[20] H Ritchie, AJ Jamieson and SB Piertney, 'Heat-Shock Protein Adaptation in Abyssal and Hadal Amphipods' (2018) 155 Deep Sea Research Part II: Topical Studies in Oceanography 61

<https://www.sciencedirect.com/science/article/pii/S096706451630315 0?utm_source=chatgpt.com> accessed 17 September 2025; Fumiyoshi Abe, 'Molecular Responses to High Hydrostatic Pressure in Eukaryotes: Genetic Insights from Studies on Saccharomyces Cerevisiae' (2021) 10 Biology 1305 <https://pmc.ncbi.nlm.nih.gov/articles/PMC8698847/> accessed 17 September 2025.

[21] Paul A Cziko and others, 'Antifreeze Protein-Induced Superheating of Ice inside Antarctic Notothenioid Fishes Inhibits Melting during Summer Warming' (2014) 111 Proceedings of the National Academy of Sciences 14583 </doi/pdf/10.1073/pnas.1410256111?download=true> accessed 17 September 2025.

[22] MJS Denny and TJ Dawson, 'Effects of Dehydration on Body-Water Distribution in Desert Kangaroos' (1975) 229 The American journal of physiology 251 <https://pubmed.ncbi.nlm.nih.gov/1147052/> accessed 17 September 2025.

[23] Karla T Moeller and others, 'Dehydration Enhances Multiple Physiological Defense Mechanisms in a Desert Lizard, Heloderma Suspectum' (2017) 220 Journal of Experimental Biology 2166 <https://dx.doi.org/10.1242/jeb.150367> accessed 17 September 2025.

[24] Anthony V. Signore and Jay F Storz, 'Biochemical Pedomorphosis and Genetic Assimilation in the Hypoxia Adaptation of Tibetan Antelope' (2020) 6 Science Advances 5447 </doi/pdf/10.1126/sciadv.abb5447?download=true> accessed 17 September 2025.

[25] Jun Bai and others, 'Genetic and Immune Changes in Tibetan High-Altitude Populations Contribute to Biological Adaptation to Hypoxia' (2022) 27 Environmental health and preventive medicine <https://pubmed.ncbi.nlm.nih.gov/36244759/> accessed 17 September 2025.

[26] BPH Righetti and others, 'Relating Diving Behavior and Antioxidant Status: Insights from Oxidative Stress Biomarkers in the Blood of Two Distinct Divers, Mirounga Leonina and Arctocephalus Australis' (2014) 173 Comparative Biochemistry and Physiology - A Molecular and Integrative Physiology 1 <https://pubmed.ncbi.nlm.nih.gov/24607367/> accessed 17 September 2025.

[27] Nadiezhda Cantú-Medellín and others, 'Differential Antioxidant Protection in Tissues from Marine Mammals with Distinct Diving Capacities. Shallow/Short vs. Deep/Long Divers' (2011) 158 Comparative Biochemistry and Physiology - A Molecular and Integrative Physiology 438 <https://pubmed.ncbi.nlm.nih.gov/21147244/> accessed 17 September 2025.

[28] Kaitlin N Allen and others, 'Hypoxia Exposure Blunts Angiogenic Signaling and Upregulates the Antioxidant System in Endothelial Cells Derived from Elephant Seals' (2024) 22 BMC Biology 1 <https://bmcbiol.biomedcentral.com/articles/10.1186/s12915-024-01892-3> accessed 17 September 2025.

[29] A Benini and SK Bonar, 'Andreas Vesalius 1514-1564' (1996) 21 Spine 1388 <https://pubmed.ncbi.nlm.nih.gov/8725935/> accessed 17 September 2025.

[30] GA Lindeboom, 'Jan Swammerdam (1637-1680) and His Biblia Naturae.' (1982) 17 Clio medica (Amsterdam, Netherlands) 113; Iain C Sutcliffe, 'Celebrating the 80th Anniversary of Antonie van Leeuwenhoek: A Special Issue' (2014) 106 Antonie van Leeuwenhoek 1 <https://pubmed.ncbi.nlm.nih.gov/24906661/> accessed 17 September 2025.

[31] D McGonagle and T Georgouli, 'The Importance of "Mechnikov's Thorn" for an Improved Understanding of 21st Century Medicine and Immunology: A View from the Eye' (2008) 68 Scandinavian journal of immunology 129 <https://pubmed.ncbi.nlm.nih.gov/18510591/> accessed 17 September 2025.

[32] JH Dirckx, 'Armand J. Quick: Pioneer and Prophet of Coagulation Research' (1980) 92 Annals of internal medicine 553 <https://pubmed.ncbi.nlm.nih.gov/6987933/> accessed 17 September 2025; Alvin H Schmaier, 'Oscar D. Ratnoff: A Man for All Seasons' (2010) 104 Thrombosis and haemostasis 863 <https://pubmed.ncbi.nlm.nih.gov/20941454/> accessed 17 September 2025.

[33] 'Lagundi: Anti-Cough and Anti-Asthma Medicine - Philippine Council for Health Research and Development' <https://www.pchrd.dost.gov.ph/heartnovation/lagundi-anti-cough-and-

anti-asthma-medicine/?utm_source=chatgpt.com> accessed 17 September 2025; Ruel Cayona and Evelyn Creencia, 'Discovery of a "Cocktail" of Potential SARS-COV-2 Main Protease Inhibitors through Virtual Screening of Known Chemical Components of Vitex Negundo L. ("Lagundi")' (2022) 18 Medicinal chemistry (Shariqah (United Arab Emirates)) 364 <https://pubmed.ncbi.nlm.nih.gov/34148541/> accessed 17 September 2025.

[34] Nurul Ain Ismail and others, 'Antimicrobial Activities and Phytochemical Properties of Blumea Balsamifera against Pathogenic Microorganisms' (2022) 15 Journal of Medicine and Life 951 <https://pmc.ncbi.nlm.nih.gov/articles/PMC9514820/> accessed 17 September 2025; 'Sambong Tablet: Herbal Drug Formulation for Kidney Stones - Philippine Council for Health Research and Development' <https://www.pchrd.dost.gov.ph/heartnovation/sambong-tablet-herbal-drug-formulation-for-kidney-stones/?utm_source=chatgpt.com> accessed 17 September 2025.

[35] Mayank Kulshreshtha and others, 'Pharmacognostical, Phytochemical and Pharmacological Aspects of Quisqualis Indica: An Update' (2018) 1 Journal of Nature and Science of Medicine 41.

[36] György Csaba, 'Hormesis and Immunity: A Review' (2019) 66 Acta microbiologica et immunologica Hungarica 155 <https://pubmed.ncbi.nlm.nih.gov/30014704/> accessed 17 September 2025.

[37] Christopher J Coates and others, 'Host Defences of Invertebrates to Pathogens and Parasites' [2022] Invertebrate Pathology 3.

[38] ROLF LUDVIGSEN, 'Rapid Repair of Traumatic Injury by an Ordovician Trilobite' (1977) 10 Lethaia 205.

[39] Tito Aureliano and others, 'Several Occurrences of Osteomyelitis in Dinosaurs from a Site in the Bauru Group, Cretaceous of Southeast Brazil' [2025] The Anatomical Record </doi/pdf/10.1002/ar.70003> accessed 17 September 2025.

[40] Asher Ornoy and Richard K Miller, 'Yolk Sac Development, Function and Role in Rodent Pregnancy' (2023) 115 Birth defects research 1243 <https://pubmed.ncbi.nlm.nih.gov/36949669/> accessed 17

September 2025; Gianluca Amadei and others, 'Embryo Model Completes Gastrulation to Neurulation and Organogenesis' (2022) 610 Nature 143 <https://pubmed.ncbi.nlm.nih.gov/36007540/> accessed 17 September 2025.

[41] Léon Sann and others, 'Serum Vitamin K1 Concentration and Vitamin K-Dependent Clotting Factor Activity in Maternal and Fetal Cord Blood' (1985) 153 American Journal of Obstetrics and Gynecology 771 <https://pubmed.ncbi.nlm.nih.gov/4073142/> accessed 17 September 2025.

[42] Elisabeth Robinson and others, 'Neutrophil Responses to RSV Infection Show Differences between Infant and Adult Neutrophils' (2024) 79 Thorax 545 <https://pubmed.ncbi.nlm.nih.gov/38050163/> accessed 17 September 2025.

[43] Ana Catarina Lunz Macedo and Lourdes Isaac, 'Systemic Lupus Erythematosus and Deficiencies of Early Components of the Complement Classical Pathway' (2016) 7 Frontiers in Immunology 55 <https://pmc.ncbi.nlm.nih.gov/articles/PMC4764694/> accessed 17 September 2025.

[44] Alberto De Zubiria Salgado and Catalina Herrera-Diaz, 'Lupus Nephritis: An Overview of Recent Findings' (2012) 2012 Autoimmune Diseases 849684 <https://pmc.ncbi.nlm.nih.gov/articles/PMC3318208/> accessed 17 September 2025.

[45] Fosca AF Di Prima and others, 'Antiphospholipid Syndrome during Pregnancy: The State of the Art' (2011) 5 Journal of Prenatal Medicine 41 <https://pmc.ncbi.nlm.nih.gov/articles/PMC3279165/> accessed 17 September 2025.

[46] Boce Song and others, 'Inflammatory Factors Driving Atherosclerotic Plaque Progression New Insights' (2022) 10 Journal of Translational Internal Medicine 36 <https://pmc.ncbi.nlm.nih.gov/articles/PMC8997796/> accessed 17 September 2025.

[47] Lejla Alic, Kristina Dendinovic and Nikolina Papac-Milicevic, 'The Complement System in Lipid-Mediated Pathologies' (2024) 15 Frontiers in Immunology 1511886 <https://pmc.ncbi.nlm.nih.gov/articles/PMC11614835/> accessed 17 September 2025.

[48] Danyaal Ain and others, 'The Role of Complement in the Tumor Microenvironment' (2021) 10 Faculty Reviews 80 <https://pmc.ncbi.nlm.nih.gov/articles/PMC8725651/> accessed 17 September 2025.

[49] Man Yan and others, 'Roles of Tumor-Associated Neutrophils in Tumor Metastasis and Its Clinical Applications' (2022) 10 Frontiers in Cell and Developmental Biology 938289 <https://pmc.ncbi.nlm.nih.gov/articles/PMC9428510/> accessed 17 September 2025.

[50] Tino Emanuele Poloni and others, 'COVID-19 Pathology in the Lung, Kidney, Heart and Brain: The Different Roles of T-Cells, Macrophages, and Microthrombosis' (2022) 11 Cells 3124 <https://pmc.ncbi.nlm.nih.gov/articles/PMC9563269/> accessed 17 September 2025.

[51] Mariana Collete and others, 'Neutrophil Extracellular Trap Markers in Post Mortem Lung Biopsies from COVID-19 Patients' (2025) 26 International Journal of Molecular Sciences 8059 <https://www.mdpi.com/1422-0067/26/16/8059/htm> accessed 17 September 2025.

[52] Paolo Macor and others, 'Multi-Organ Complement Deposition in COVID-19 Patients' [2021] medRxiv 2021.01.07.21249116 <https://www.medrxiv.org/content/10.1101/2021.01.07.21249116v1> accessed 17 September 2025.

[53] WS Fields, 'The History of Leeching and Hirudin' (1991) 21 Suppl 1 Haemostasis 3 <https://pubmed.ncbi.nlm.nih.gov/1894194/> accessed 17 September 2025.

[54] Gregory Tsoucalas and others, 'Historical Hallmarks of Anticoagulation and Antiplatelet Agents' (2016) 22 Current pharmaceutical design 1857 <https://pubmed.ncbi.nlm.nih.gov/26750139/> accessed 17 September 2025.

[55] Frank Misselwitz, Scott D Berkowitz and Elisabeth Perzborn, 'The Discovery and Development of Rivaroxaban' (2011) 1222 Annals of the New York Academy of Sciences 64 <https://pubmed.ncbi.nlm.nih.gov/21434944/> accessed 17 September 2025.

[56] Xuan Yuan and others, ‘Small-Molecule Factor D Inhibitors Selectively Block the Alternative Pathway of Complement in Paroxysmal Nocturnal Hemoglobinuria and Atypical Hemolytic Uremic Syndrome’ (2017) 102 Haematologica 466 <https://haematologica.org/article/view/7998> accessed 17 September 2025; Blanca Tarragon Estebanez and Andrew S Bomback, ‘C3 Glomerulopathy: Novel Treatment Paradigms’ (2024) 9 Kidney International Reports 569 <https://www.sciencedirect.com/science/article/pii/S2468024923016297> accessed 17 September 2025.

[57] Melissa Meyer, ‘Thicker than Water: The Origins of Blood as Symbol and Ritual’ [2005] Thicker Than Water: The Origins of Blood as Symbol and Ritual 1.

[58] MY Nabofa, ‘Blood Symbolism in African Religion’ (1985) 21 Religious Studies 389 <https://www.cambridge.org/core/journals/religious-studies/article/abs/blood-symbolism-in-african-religion/376A48204A853F40E3E4ED3B931E15CF> accessed 17 September 2025; Ian Watts, ‘Blood Symbolism at the Root of Symbolic Culture? African Hunter-Gatherer Perspectives’ (2024) 76 Journal of Anthropological Archaeology 101627 <https://www.sciencedirect.com/science/article/pii/S0278416524000588?utm_source=chatgpt.com> accessed 17 September 2025.

[59] ‘Tryals Proposed by Mr. Boyle to Dr. Lower, to Be Made by Him, for the Improvement of Tranfusing Blood out of One Live Animal into Another; Promised Numb. 20. p. 357’ (1665) 1 Philosophical Transactions of the Royal Society of London 385.

[60] Haoqiang He and others, ‘Xue-Fu-Zhu-Yu Capsule in the Treatment of Qi Stagnation and Blood Stasis Syndrome: A Study Protocol for a Randomised Controlled Pilot and Feasibility Trial’ (2018) 19 Trials 515 <https://pmc.ncbi.nlm.nih.gov/articles/PMC6151047/> accessed 17 September 2025.

[61] Naomi Janowitz, ‘Rereading Sacrifice: The Semiosis of Blood’ (2015) 3 Signs and Society 193 <https://www.cambridge.org/core/journals/signs-and-society/article/rereading-sacrifice-the-semiosis-of-

blood/57CC9DC468A990956AC6AE1EAE7679FB> accessed 17 September 2025.

[62] Nobuo Okumura, Oleg V. Gorkun and Susan T Lord, 'Severely Impaired Polymerization of Recombinant Fibrinogen γ-364 Asp → His, the Substitution Discovered in a Heterozygous Individual' (1997) 272 Journal of Biological Chemistry 29596 <https://pubmed.ncbi.nlm.nih.gov/9368024/> accessed 17 September 2025.

[63] Sarah E Stabenfeldt and others, 'Engineering Fibrin Polymers through Engagement of Alternative Polymerization Mechanisms' (2012) 33 Biomaterials 535 <https://pubmed.ncbi.nlm.nih.gov/22018389/> accessed 17 September 2025.

[64] Natalie Smith and others, 'Identification and Characterization of Novel Mutations Implicated in Congenital Fibrinogen Disorders' (2018) 2 Research and Practice in Thrombosis and Haemostasis 800 </doi/pdf/10.1002/rth2.12127> accessed 17 September 2025.

[65] Judith J De Vries and others, 'Effects of Post-Translational Modifications of Fibrinogen on Clot Formation, Clot Structure, and Fibrinolysis: A Systematic Review' (2020) 40 Arteriosclerosis, thrombosis, and vascular biology 554 <https://pubmed.ncbi.nlm.nih.gov/31914791/> accessed 17 September 2025.

[66] Alexandra H Antonioli and others, 'Modulation of the Alternative Pathway of Complement by Murine Factor H-Related Proteins' (2017) 200 Journal of immunology (Baltimore, Md.: 1950) 316 <https://pmc.ncbi.nlm.nih.gov/articles/PMC5736413/> accessed 17 September 2025.

[67] V Michael Holers, 'The Complement System as a Therapeutic Target in Autoimmunity' (2003) 107 Clinical Immunology 140 <https://pubmed.ncbi.nlm.nih.gov/12804527/> accessed 17 September 2025; B Paul Morgan and Claire L Harris, 'Complement Therapeutics; History and Current Progress' (2003) 40 Molecular Immunology 159 <https://pubmed.ncbi.nlm.nih.gov/12914822/> accessed 17 September 2025.

[68] Sydney J Stine and others, 'Exosome and Biomimetic Nanoparticle Therapies for Cardiac Regenerative Medicine' (2020) 15 Current stem cell

research & therapy 674 <https://pubmed.ncbi.nlm.nih.gov/32148200/> accessed 17 September 2025; Michael Sun and others, 'Direct Delivery of Plasmin Using Clot-Anchoring Thrombin-Responsive Nanoparticles for Targeted Fibrinolytic Therapy' (2022) 21 Journal of thrombosis and haemostasis: JTH 983 <https://pmc.ncbi.nlm.nih.gov/articles/PMC10148984/> accessed 17 September 2025.

[69] Karina Pombo García and others, 'Zwitterionic-Coated "Stealth" Nanoparticles for Biomedical Applications: Recent Advances in Countering Biomolecular Corona Formation and Uptake by the Mononuclear Phagocyte System' (2014) 10 Small (Weinheim an der Bergstrasse, Germany) 2516 <https://pubmed.ncbi.nlm.nih.gov/24687857/> accessed 17 September 2025; Benjamin M King and Jennifer Fiegel, 'Zwitterionic Polymer Coatings Enhance Gold Nanoparticle Stability and Uptake in Various Biological Environments' (2022) 24 The AAPS journal <https://pubmed.ncbi.nlm.nih.gov/34984558/> accessed 17 September 2025.

[70] Haichun Li and others, 'Size Dependency of Circulation and Biodistribution of Biomimetic Nanoparticles: Red Blood Cell Membrane-Coated Nanoparticles' (2019) 8 Cells 881 <https://pmc.ncbi.nlm.nih.gov/articles/PMC6721642/> accessed 17 September 2025; Ashley V. Kroll, Ronnie H Fang and Liangfang Zhang, 'Biointerfacing and Applications of Cell Membrane-Coated Nanoparticles' (2016) 28 Bioconjugate chemistry 23 <https://pmc.ncbi.nlm.nih.gov/articles/PMC5471317/> accessed 17 September 2025.

[71] Donghui Zhu, 'Mathematical Modeling of Blood Coagulation Cascade: Kinetics of Intrinsic and Extrinsic Pathways in Normal and Deficient Conditions' (2007) 18 Blood coagulation & fibrinolysis: an international journal in haemostasis and thrombosis 637 <https://pubmed.ncbi.nlm.nih.gov/17890951/> accessed 17 September 2025.

[72] Christian Tokarski and others, 'Agent-Based Modeling Approach of Immune Defense against Spores of Opportunistic Human Pathogenic Fungi' (2012) 3 Frontiers in microbiology <https://pubmed.ncbi.nlm.nih.gov/22557995/> accessed 17 September 2025.

[73] Nehemiah Zewde and others, 'Quantitative Modeling of the Alternative Pathway of the Complement System' (2016) 11 PloS one <https://pubmed.ncbi.nlm.nih.gov/27031863/> accessed 17 September 2025.

[74] Mark GE. Kelly and Michel Foucault, 'Foucault's History of Sexuality. Volume 1, The Will to Knowledge' 192; Michel Foucault and others, 'Lecture Eleven' [2003] Society must be defended: lectures at the Collège de France, 1975-76 xxiii <http://www.loc.gov/catdir/toc/hol031/2002074998.html%5Cnhttp://www.loc.gov/catdir/description/hol031/2002074998.html> accessed 17 September 2025.

Did you love *Currents of Protection*? Then you should read *Hiyang: Pilipinong Pananaw ng Parmakohenetika* by Brian Pollo!

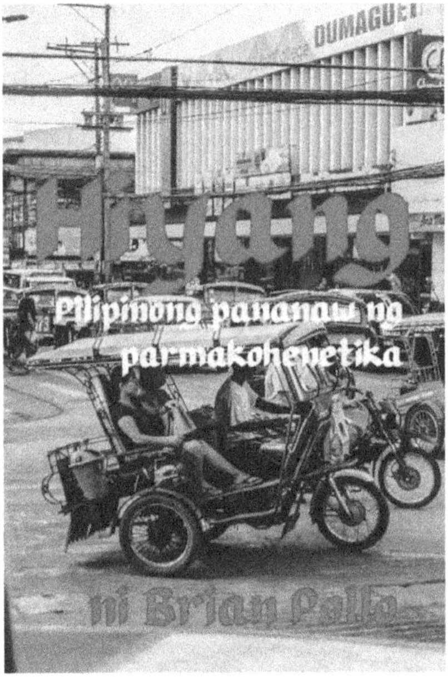

In everyday Filipino life, the word *hiyang* carries profound meaning. A person might say, "*hiyang sa akin ang gamot na ito*" (*i.e.,* this medicine suits me) or lament that a treatment is "*hindi hiyang*." For generations, Filipinos have used this term to capture the mystery of why some remedies work for certain people but not for others. What once seemed like cultural intuition is now at the center of a rapidly advancing science: pharmacogenetics.

Pharmacogenetics is the study of how our genes influence drug response. It explains why two patients given the same dose of the same medicine may experience very different results: healing in one, side effects in another, or no effect at all. What Filipino families have long described through *hiyang*, science now investigates through enzymes, genetic variants, and molecular pathways. This book builds a bridge between these worlds, showing that cultural wisdom and modern research are not enemies but partners in understanding human health.

Across its chapters, the book introduces the fundamentals of pharmacogenetics in clear, accessible language. Readers learn about genetic polymorphisms in enzymes such as CYP450 and their impact on drug metabolism. They discover how pharmacogenetic testing guides treatment choices in cardiovascular disease, infectious diseases, and oncology. Alongside the science, the text interweaves stories and expressions of *hiyang*, illustrating how Filipinos have long recognized the principle that "not all medicines fit all people."

Beyond the technical, the book raises questions at the intersection of ethics, culture, and medicine. What are the implications of pharmacogenetic testing in resource-limited settings? How can indigenous concepts like *hiyang* enrich global health conversations and promote cultural humility among practitioners? How do we ensure that advances in precision medicine remain accessible and equitable, rather than widening gaps in care?

This is not just a scientific primer but also a cultural exploration. It speaks to physicians, pharmacists, students, and researchers who wish to understand pharmacogenetics in a broader human context. It also invites general readers to reflect on how everyday language encodes valuable insights into health. By situating *hiyang* within the global movement toward personalized medicine, the book offers a uniquely Filipino contribution to a universal challenge: making healthcare more precise, more personal, and more just.

Ultimately, this book argues that healing has always been about finding the right fit, between person and medicine, between genes and treatment, between culture and science. *Hiyang* is more than a word; it is a bridge. And by crossing it, we discover new ways of thinking about medicine, identity, and the shared search for well-being in a diverse and interconnected world.

Read more at https://sites.google.com/view/brian-pollo/home.

Also by Brian Pollo

Hiyang: Pilipinong Pananaw ng Parmakohenetika
Hiyang: Pilipinong Pananaw ng Parmakohenetika
Salinlunas: Natural Products & Pharmacognosy
Salinlunas: Natural Products & Pharmacognosy
Currents of Protection
Currents of Protection
Resistance Rising: Genetics, Evolution, and the Future of Infectious Diseases
Resistance Rising: Genetics, Evolution, and the Future of Infectious Diseases
Phonies: Authenticity Performance Fakery
Phonies: Authenticity Performance Fakery
Biographies in Blood: The Making of Medical Modernity and Asian Medical Innovations

Watch for more at https://sites.google.com/view/brian-pollo/home.

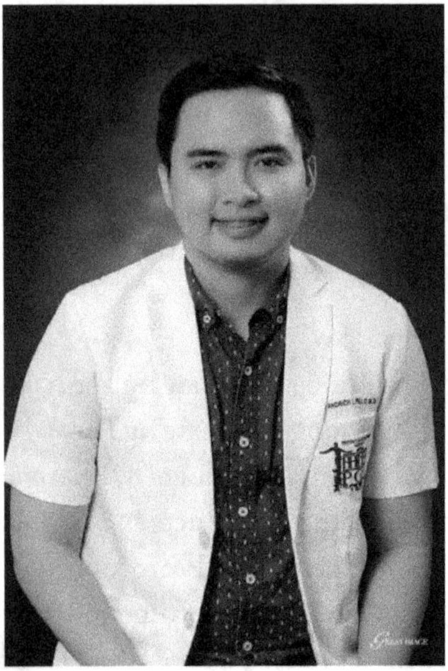

About the Author

Brian Pollo is an MD-PhD candidate, educator, and writer whose work spans biochemistry, ethnomedicine, and the history of science. They study how complement, coagulation, and innate immunity adapt in extreme environments, while also tracing the cultural and symbolic roles of blood in human storytelling. Their writing blends scientific rigor with narrative inquiry, reflecting a commitment to both biomedical innovation and the preservation of ancestral knowledge.

Read more at https://sites.google.com/view/brian-pollo/home.

About the Publisher

Sandiwà Publishing is an independent press devoted to works that unite spirit (*diwà*) and intellect. Its catalogue bridges creative nonfiction, ethnomedicine, history, and the sciences, reflecting the conviction that knowledge is strongest when culture and inquiry walk together. Each publication honors heritage while engaging the challenges of the present, affirming that literature can be both an archive of memory and a spark for new ideas.

Read more at https://sites.google.com/view/brian-pollo/home.

www.ingramcontent.com/pod-product-compliance
Lightning Source LLC
LaVergne TN
LVHW022102200926
848481LV00003B/1031